Dysglycemic Pedal Zymosis: Orthodox vs Corpuscular Moneric Denotation and Quantism

Aura Lux

Dysglycemic Pedal Zymosis: Orthodox vs Corpuscular Moneric Denotation and Quantism

First Edition August 2025

Written by Aura Lux

TABLE OF CONTENTS

Page No.

LIST OF TABLES

LIST OF FIGURES

LIST OF ABBREVIATIONS

ABI	:	Ankle Brachial Index
ADA	:	American Diabetes Association
ADES	:	Amrita Diabetes and Epidemiological Survey
AER	:	Albumin Excretion Rate
AGE	:	Advanced Glycation End Product
BA	:	Blood Agar
BEC	:	Bio-ethical Committee
BHI	:	Brain Heart Infusion
BMI	:	Body Mass Index
bps	:	Base Pairs
CVD	:	Cardiovascular Disease
CAD	:	Cardioarterial Disease
CLSI	:	Clinical and Laboratory Standards Institutes
cm^2	:	Centimeter Square
CRP	:	C-Reactive Protein
CURES	:	Chennai Urban Rural Epidemiology Study
DAG	:	Diacyl Glycerol
DCCT	:	Diabetes Control and Complication Trial
DFI	:	Diabetic Foot Infection
DFU	:	Diabetic Foot Ulcers
DGGE	:	Denaturing Gradient Gel Electrophoresis
DM	:	Diabetes Mellitus
DNA	:	Deoxy-Ribo-Nucleic Acid
EDTA	:	Ethylene-Di-Amine-Tetra Acetic Acid
eGFR	:	Estimated Glomerular Filteration Rate
ELISA	:	Enzyme Linked Immunosorbent Assay
eNOS	:	Endothelial Nitric Oxide Synthase 3
ESKD	:	End Stage Kidney Disease
GDM	:	Gestational Diabetes Mellitus
HbA1c	:	Glycated Hemoglobin
HDL-C	:	High Density Lipoprotein Cholesterol
HLA	:	Human Leukocyte Antigen

HLAp	:	Human Leukocyte Antigen
HMP	:	Hexosamine Phosphate Shunt
HRP	:	Horseradish Peroxidase
ICMR	:	Indian Council of Medical Research
IDDM	:	Insulin Dependent Diabetes Mellitus
IDF	:	International Diabetes Federation
IDSA	:	Infectious Disease Society of America
IEC	:	Institutional Ethical Committee
IGF	:	Insulin-like Growth Factor
IL-1	:	Interleukin-1
IL-6	:	Interleukin-6
IV	:	Intravenous
IWGDF	:	International Working Group on the Diabetic Foot
kPa	:	Kilo Pascal
LDL-C	:	Low-Density Lipoprotein Cholesterol
mg/dL	:	Milligram/Deciliter
MHA	:	Mueller Hilton Agar
MHC	:	Major Histocompatibility Complex
mM	:	Milimolar
mmol/L	:	Milimole/Litre
mmol/mol	:	milimolar/mole
MODY	:	Maturity onset- Diabetes of Young
MRSA	:	Methicillin Resistant *Staphylococcus aureus*
NA	:	Nutrient Agar
NADPH	:	Nictonamide Adenine Dinucleotide Dinucleotide Phosphate
NO	:	Nitric Oxide
NPDR	:	Non-proliferative Diabetic retinopathy
PAD	:	Peripheral Arterial Disease
PAI-1	:	Plasminogen Activator Inhibitor-1
PCR	:	Polymerase Chain Reaction
PDGF	:	Platelet Derive Growth Factor
pKC	:	Protein Kinase-C
PPDR	:	Pre-Proliferative Diabetic Retinopathy

RAGES	:	Receptors of Advanced Glycation End Products
RANTES	:	Regulated on Activation, Normal T Cell Expressed and Secreted
ROS	:	Reactive Oxygen Species
T1DM	:	Type 1 Diabetes Mellitus
T2DM	:	Type 2 Diabetes Mellitus
TAE	:	Tris-acetate-EDTA
TGF-β-1	:	Transforming growth factor beta -1
TIA	:	Transient Ischemic Attack
TMB	:	3,3',5,5'-Tetramethylbenzidine
TNF-α	:	Tumor Necrosis Factor
UDP	:	Uridine-di-phosphate-Glucose
μgm	:	Microgram
Ml	:	Mircolitre
UTSA	:	University of Texas Classification System
VEGF	:	Vascular Endothelial Growth Factor
VLDL	:	Very Low Density Lipoprotein
WHO	:	World Health Organization
WNL	:	Within Normal Limit

Introduction

1. INTRODUCTION:

Diabetes mellitus (DM) is considered as one of the major burden in health care systems and is now a global epidemic threat that has amplified several folds over the past 2 decades. Over the past three decades, the global burden of DM has swelled from 30 million in 1985 to 382 million in 2014, with current trends indicating that these rates will only continue to rise (Wild et al., 2004). The latest estimates by the International Diabetes Federation (IDF) projects that 592 million worldwide will have DM by 2035. In India, about 50.8 million subjects are suffering from DM, which is expected to rise to 87 million by 2030 (Shaw et al., 2011).

Patients with DM are prone to development of multiple secondary complications. The complications associated with DM are macrovascular (due to damage to large blood vessels) or microvascular (due to damage to small blood vessels). The microvascular complications includes damage to eyes (retinopathy) causing blindness, to nerves (neuropathy) causing diabetic foot ulcers (DFUs) and subsequent amputation in severe infection, and to kidneys (nephropathy) leading to renal failure. Large prospective clinical analysis has reported a strong interrelationship between hyperglycemia and microvascular complications in patients with DM (DCCT., 1993; UKPDS., 1998). The hyperglycemia in DM is also linked to accelerated atheroscelerotic macrovascular disorders affecting blood supply to vital organs such as brain, heart, and lower limbs (Cade., 2008). The condition pathogically is similar to vascular disorders in nondiabetics, but is more progressive and extensive in diabetic subjects (Ras-Mandsen et al., 2013). The overall risk of cardiovascular complications is increased by two to six fold in diabetic subjects.

Amalgamation of accelerated lower extremity arterial disease and neuropathy, DM accounts for about 50% of non-traumatic limb loss in United States (Resnick et al., 1999). DFUs which are a common problem of DM have shown an increasing drift since many decades. Studies report that in total, 15% of patients with diabetes suffer from DFU during their lifetime and about 28% of them may undergo some form of amputation or lower limb loss (Boulton et al., 2005; Reiber et al., 1998). Foot ulcer is a common complication of both type 1 and type 2 diabetics (Boulton., 2000). DFU is considered as a major source of substantial increase in morbidity and a foremost reason for hospitalization in patients with DM. Indeed, DFU can lead to infection, systemic toxicity, gangrene, lower extremity amputations, and eventually death if proper treatment and care is not provided. About 85% of subjects with DFUs undergo amputations (Pendsey et al., 2010). Furthermore, DFU is responsible for extensive physical and emotional suffering as well as financial losses that lower the quality of life. At least 40% of lower limb losses in diabetic patients can be prevented with a managed team approach to wound care (Lavery et al., 1998).

Diabetic foot ulcerations results from interaction of a number of component causes, none of which as single is sufficient to cause ulcers, but when combined complete the casual pathway to skin breakdown (Pendsey eta al., 2010). Many risk factors are responsible for development of DFUs such as gender (more frequently in males), longer duration of diabetes (>10 years), older age of patients, high Body Mass Index (BMI), and other co-morbidities such as peripheral neuropathy, peripheral vascular disease (PVD), raised glycated hemoglobin level (HbA1c), high plantar pressures, foot deformities, infections, and inappropriate foot self-care habits (Armstrong et al., 1998; Boyko et al., 1999; Pecoraro et al., 1990). Although infection is rarely implicated in the etiology of DFUs, the ulcers are susceptible to infection once the lesion develops. Infection in DFUs is a common, complex and costly problem causing severe co-morbidities and responsible for largest number of diabetes-related hospital bed days (Reiber et al., 1996) and most proximate reason of amputations (Reiber et al., 1999). A multi-centric study attributed 63 percent of DFUs to the clinical triad of peripheral sensory neuropathy, trauma, and deformity (Reiber et al., 1999).

The three major aspects of neuropathy i.e. sensory, motor, and autonomic contribute to ulcerations in foot. Sensory neuropathy causes sensation loss thereby reducing the perception of painful, thermal and vibration mobilities, and trauma/injury. Motor neuropathy leads to disturbances of foot posture, weakness and wasting of muscles of the foot causing imbalances between flexor and extensor muscles resulting in clawing of toes, prominent metatarsal heads and arch flattering. This leads to bearing the body's weight by smaller areas-typically the metatarsals heads and the heat and extensive pressure loading at these points stimulate the callus formation which is a precursor of ulceration (Robinson et al., 1992; Sosenko et al., 1986). Autonomic neuropathy leads to sudomotor function and atypical blood supply to soles of feet. With deportation in functions of sweat and sebaceous glands of foot, skin becomes dry and keratinizes which cracks and fissures more frequently, making a portal for infection.

PVD in isolation is rarely involved in the pathogenesis of DFUs. However, a combination of atherosclerotic peripheral arteries along with minor injury and subsequent infection increases the blood demand beyond the circulation limits, causing ischemic diabetic foot lesions. Doppler-based ankle pressure assessment can be falsely high in subjects with long-standing diabetes, but the presence or absence of a dorsal pedis or posterior tibial is a non-invasive and simplest indicator of significant ischemia.

Most of the injuries on feet of diabetic patients with neuropathy occur on forefoot with equal distribution on dorsal and plantar aspects, and those on plantar surface occur at high-pressure areas (Veves et al., 1991; Stess et al., 1986). According to plantar pressure examination defined by Armstrong et al., 1998, pressure value of 750 kPa will provide a cut-off value to differentiate between patients with high and low risk of ulcerations. The second major factor is foot deformity which is more likely a key factor of injury on foot. Higher foot pressure on dorsal and plantar regions will lead to many skin injuries. One of the strongest predictors of ulceration is a previous ulcer or amputation of another leg. Imbalances caused in flexor and extensor muscles leads to foot deformities like clawing of toes, prominent metatarsal heads. In turn, combination of foot deformities along with proprioceptive loss due to neuropathy leads to increase in the pressure and load under diabetic foot (Brownlee et al., 2003). In Charcot foot deformity, the surface of foot is erythematous, swollen and hot. Another important aspect is the callus formation in foot. The limited mobility in joints also plays an important risk factor in development of foot ulcers in diabetics. Delbridge et al., 1985, reported the relationship between limited joint mobility and ulcers on plantar region. Previous ulceration or amputation of another leg is also considered as strongest predictors of foot ulcers. Patients suffering from other secondary complications such as retinopathy, neuropathy is at increased risk of foot lesions, most probably reflecting widespread microvascular damage. Several studies reported that patients with poor understanding of diabetes and its management are more prone to ulcerations (Reiber et al., 1992).

Diabetic foot infection (DFI) is defined as any infra-malleolar infection in patient with DM (Lipsky et al., 2004). The spectrum of infection may include superficial cellulitis, myositis abscesses, necrotizing fasciitis, septic arthritis, tendinitis, and osteomyelitis. The diabetic wound is a result of complicated amalgam of potential risk factors (Caputo et al., 1994; Frykberg, 1998) because, once the protective layer of skin is breached, underlying tissues are exposed to bacterial colonization. The infection in active state can be contiguous and may involve deeper tissues. However, in ischemic limbs, the infection worsens rapidly. The sequence of events can be rapid (occurring within hours or days), especially in ischemic limb. The immunological disturbances, especially involving polymorphonuclear leukocytes, may affect patients with DM, thereby increasing the risk and severity of foot infection (Schubert et al., 1995; Gin., 1993; Joshi et al., 1990). These have ranged from highlighting the occurrence of particular species (Schraibman., 1990) or group of organisms (Wall et al., 2002) to assessing the impact of microbial populations on clinical outcomes.

The treatment of infection in diabetic patient is difficult. The information regarding the etiological factors is needed in the selection of definitive antibiotic therapy. Cellulitis is the most easily treatable and reversible form of foot infections in diabetics. However, infection of deeper tissues are usually curable, but can be life-threatening and may lead to substantial long-term morbidity (Frykberg., 1999). The incidence of infection-related co-morbidities such as incidence of major limb amputation (Armstrong et al., 1995; Calhoun et al., 1988) can be reduced by optimal management. Available published evidence does not support the use of antibiotics for management of clinically uninfected lesions either to enhance wound healing or as prophylaxis against infection (Chantealu et al., 1996; Hirsch et al., 1992). Antibiotic use encourages antimicrobial resistance; increases financial cost, and may cause drug-related adverse effects. In some circumstances, it is difficult to decide whether a chronic wound is infected, such as when the foot is ischemic, has abnormal coloration, or a fetid odor has friable granulation tissue, is associated with unexpected pain or tenderness, or when an otherwise properly treated ulcer fails to slow healing progress (Cutting et al., 1994; Schultz et al., 2003).

The prevalence of pathogens is variable in DFI. There are various aspects of wound microbiology responsible for the development of infected foot lesions including microbial load, diversity of microbes, and existence of infective organisms along with synergistic association amongst microbial species. Several microorganisms have been evaluated in microbial etiology of infected foot ulcers. These ranges from fungi to aerobic, and anaerobic species (Gadepalli et al., 2006; Zubair et al., 2011). The microbiology of foot ulcers is usually polymicrobial, and recent studies using molecular techniques have emphasized the complex etiology of these wounds (Davies et al., 2003).

The selection of antibiotic regime initially involves decisions about the specific drugs to be administered, the route of therapy, the spectrum of microorganisms to be covered, and involves choosing the definitive regime along with the duration of treatment. Initial therapy is usually empirical and is based on the severity of the infection and on any available microbiological data, such as recent culture and antimicrobial sensitivity. For severe or chronic infections, it is safe to commence therapy with broad-spectrum agents. These should have activity against gram-positive cocci [including Methicillin-resistant *Staphylococcus aureus* (MRSA)], as well as gram-negative and obligate anaerobic organisms (Lipsky et al., 2012). Several antibiotic trials involving patients with complicated DFIs have been conducted. The lack of standardization among makes the comparison of outcomes of different regimes inappropriate. Currently, no specific antibiotic regime has proven superior for treating these DFIs. The differing definitions of infection severity and clinical endpoints used in these publications highlights the need to develop a consensus classification system for future studies. On the basis of available studies, no single drug or combination of agents appears to be superior to others (Lipsky et al., 1999), although the available data do not allow us to recommend any specific antibiotic regime for DFI.

Infected DFU imposes a serious health stress; hence identification of causative pathogens is essential. The methodologies used in bacterial identification, therefore, play an important role. It is a well-known fact that patients with DM and foot ulcers with infection impose a serious problem despite of all preventive measures. Hence, it becomes necessary to isolate the causative microorganism in DFIs for appropriate treatment (Joseph et al., 2010). There are majorly four techniques being used for sample collection from wound of diabetic foot patients which includes aspiration, swab, tissue biopsy and curettage (Mackowiak et al., 1978). Tissue biopsy is known as the most advantageous and standard method according to several studies. But due to fear of spreading of infection, loss of adjacent structure in limb and ischemia, tissue biopsy is not advisable (Mackkowiak et al., 1978). Swab cultures are manageable since sample collection becomes easier and can be taken from any kind of wound. However, swab cultures are sometimes not reliable since it generally includes the colonizers and not the causative pathogen (Sapico et al., 1984). Even now results of swab cultures are being widely used for identification of causative microbe and selection of antibiotic. Culturing technique, therefore, plays a crucial role in identification. The identification of wound microflora by conventional approaches is based on traditional bacteriological methods (Eriksson et al., 1984). These methods depend upon the microbial growth and metabolic status and preferred in clinical diagnostic because of low cost and ease of use (Noor et al., 2015). Improving the methods of microbial diagnosis and identification may manifest in progressive wound healing. Tools of molecular biology provides powerful means to define chronic wound microbial communities. Microbiota diversity in wounds of patients can be more easily and sensitively explored by using molecular techniques than culture methodologies.

Various studies reported that a large number of microorganisms that are fastidious or nonculturable in traditional conventional methods were also revealed by PCR (Bowler et al., 1999; Dowd et al., 2008). In diabetic wounds with polymicrobial or complex bacterial isolates, it becomes technically difficult to isolate and identify more than three to six species because of different concentrations of various species and interspecies competition. Molecular techniques can also define patterns of genetic and protein expression under different clinical and morphological conditions. Molecular approaches make possible the detection of microbes without the time required for growth and environmental selection pressures inherent in the culturing process. There are only few published reports covering this aspect (Dowd et al., 2008). Furthermore, no molecular study regarding the occurrence detection of common bacterial isolates is published from northern India. However, there is paucity of data on the current aspect from Indian hospitals on the identification of bacterial isolates.

Objectives of the present study:

In view of paucity of information as outlined above, the present study was proposed to cover the following aspects.

1. A systemic evaluation and etiological study of patients with DFUs.

2. To determine the clinical and demographical variables with confounding role in pathogenesis of diabetic foot ulcers.

3. Microbial profiling and antibiotic susceptibility testing of organisms isolated from DFUs using conventional bacteriological methods.

4. Exploring the common microbial flora in pus samples from DFUs by polymerase chain reaction (PCR).

5. To establish a guideline for early laboratory diagnosis of infections and to evaluate the outcome of these studies.

6. To estimate the serum levels of immunological markers in Diabetic Foot Subjects.

2. REVIEW OF LITERATURE:

Diabetes mellitus is a group of metabolic disorders and a chronic hormonal condition, characterized by hyperglycemia due to lack of insulin production by pancreas (insulin deficiency) or when insulin is ineffective (insulin resistance) or both (ADA, 2004). All types of diabetes, both inherited and acquired, are defined by hyperglycemic state due to a relative or absolute lack of insulin, followed by development of diabetes-specific microvascular pathology in the retina, renal capillaries, and nerves of peripheries. Diabetes is also related with macrovascular comorbodities with early and accelerated atherogenesis affecting arteries that supply blood to the heart, brain, and lower limbs (Cade et al., 2008). Pathologically, this situation resembles macrovascular disease in non-diabetic patients, but it is more encapsulating and progresses more rapidly in diabetic subjects. As a consequence of the microvascular pathology, DM is now the foremost grounds of new blindness in people between age of 20-74 years and end-stage-kidney-disease (ESKD). The average life expectancy of patients with diabetic ESKD is not more than 3-4 years (Ghaderian et al., 2015) People with DM are the fastest growing group of kidney dialysis and transplant recipients (Stevens et al., 2010). Diabetes and)its associated secondary complications are a major cause of morbidity and mortality. Therefore, the life expectancy is about 7-10 years lesser than for subjects without DM because of increased mortality due to diabetic complications (Skyler., 1996). Large prospective clinical studies show a strong relationship between glycemia and diabetic microvascular complications in both type 1 diabetes mellitus (T1DM) and type 2 diabetes mellitus (T2DM) (DCCT 1993; UKPDS 1998). There is a continuous, not linear, relationship between level of glycemia and the risk of development and progression of these complications.

2.1. Epidemiology of Diabetes:

2.1.1. Global Scenario

Diabetes in all its forms imposes unacceptably high human, social and economic burden on countries at all income levels. It is described as the "*global epidemic*" of the 21st century; the rising prevalence of DM places a strong strain on resources and brings suffering to many, if the preventive measures are not put into effect. The changes in lifestyle, life expectancy and lack of information in healthcare are in part accountable for the astounding increase in the diabetes mellitus incidences. As a result, there is an upward trend of incidence, especially in industrialized urban areas. Several previous estimates of the prevalence of diabetes have been made. Whiting et al., 2011, estimated the prevalence of diabetes from data of 216 countries. They considered only 91 countries, in which studies on prevalence have been commenced, in which 5 of the 10 world's highest national prevalence occurred in the Middle-East region. The last 30 years have seen a worldwide rising tide of metabolic diseases triggered by changing lifestyle. Diabetes has traditionally been viewed as a disease of rich countries. Studies on the prevalence of diabetes mellitus around the globe are increasing and reporting a huge percentage of undiagnosed diabetes in the worldwide population. According to the estimates of World Health Organization (WHO), the high plasma glucose is the third uppermost risk factor for premature mortality, after high blood pressure and tobacco intake. IDF most recent estimates indicate that 8.8% of adults ~415 million people worldwide (aged 20-79 years), have diabetes, and the number of individuals with the disease is expected to rise beyond 642 million by 2040. Studies on the prevalence of diabetes mellitus around the globe are increasing and reporting a huge percentage of undiagnosed diabetes in the worldwide population. Among 193 million of cases currently undiagnosed, an enormous amount of individuals with diabetes is progressing towards complications unawares. Moreover, about 80% of the total number affected, dwells in low- and middle-income countries, where the epidemic is gathering pace at alarming rates. In high-income countries, approximately 87% to 91% of all people with diabetes are estimated to have type 2 diabetes, 7% with 12% of subjects are likely to have T1DM and 1% to 3% to have other types of diabetes. In developing countries, the majority of people suffering from diabetes belongs to the age group of 45 to 64 years, and by 2030, it is expected that the number of people with diabetes >64 years of age will be >82 million in developing countries and >48 million in developed countries (Tesfaye et al., 2016).

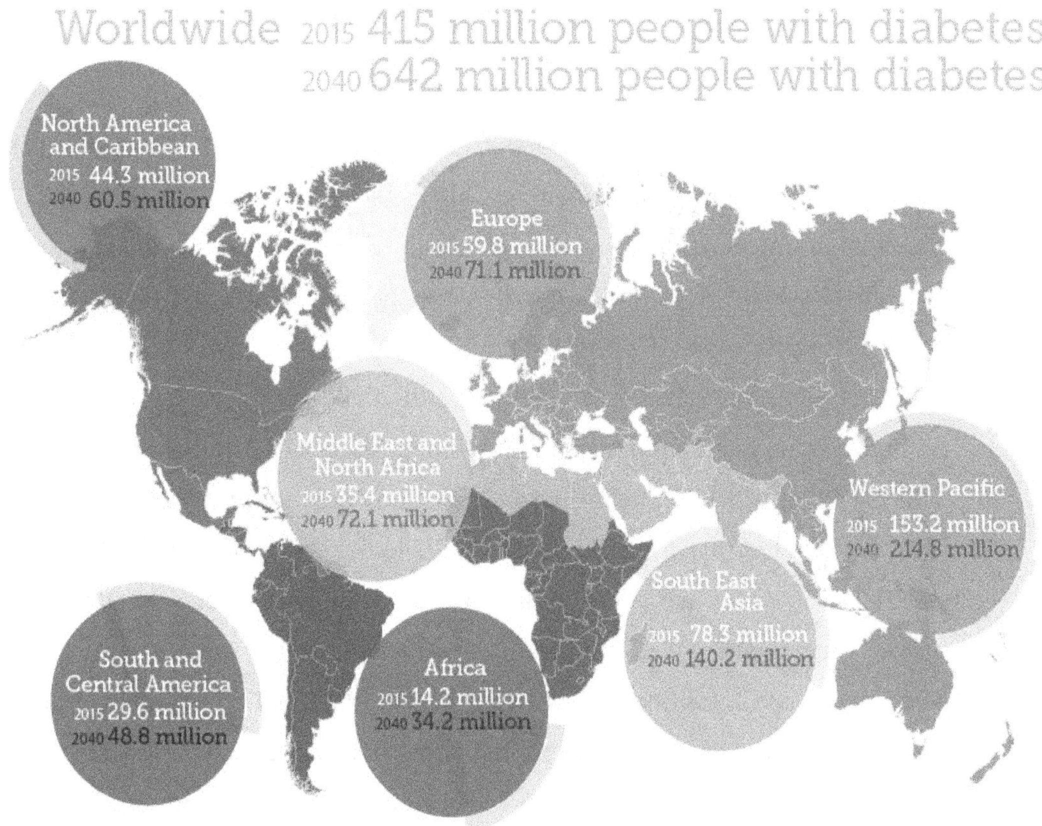

Figure 1: Prevalence of Diabetes Mellitus worldwide
(**Source:** International Diabetes Federation (IDF), 2015)

Table 1: Top 10 countries for diabetes prevalence (20-79 years), in 2013 and 2035. (IDF Diabetes Atlas/Sixth Edition).

	Country	2013 Millions		Country	2035 Millions
1	China	98.4	**1**	China	142.7
2	India	65.1	**2**	India	109.0
3	USA	24.4	**3**	USA	29.7
4	Brazil	11.9	**4**	Brazil	19.2
5	Russia	10.9	**5**	Mexico	15.7
6	Mexico	8.7	**6**	Indonesia	14.1
7	Indonesia	8.5	**7**	Egypt	13.1
8	Germany	7.6	**8**	Pakistan	12.8
9	Egypt	7.5	**9**	Turkey	11.8
10	Japan	7.2	**10**	Russia	11.2

2.1.2. National Scenario

DM in India shows the scary value of >62 million diabetic individuals (Joshi et al., 2007; Kumar et al., 2013). In the year 2000, India topped the outmost position with 31.7 million people with DM among other countries around the globe followed by China (20.8 million) and the United States (17.7 million) on second and third position respectively. Wild et al., 2004, clearly state the prevalence of DM to double globally from 171 million in 2020 to 366 million in 2030 with a maximum number of incidence in India. The predicted figure of diabetics in 2030 includes India (79.4 million), China (42.3 million) and the United States (30.3 million) (Wild et al., 2004; Whiting et al., 2011). Preliminary results obtained from a large population-based study conducted by Indian Council of Medical Research (ICMR), New Delhi, revealed that lower mass of population is affected by diabetes in states of Northern India, Chandigarh (0.12 million), Jharkhand (0.96 million) as compared to Maharashtra (9.2 million) and Tamil Nadu (4.8 million) (Anjana et al., 2011). National Urban Survey of metropolitan cities in India revealed the statistical figure of 11.7% in Kolkata (Eastern India), 6.1% in Kashmir Valley (Northern India) (Zargar et al., 2000), 11.6% in New Delhi (Northern India), 9.3% in Mumbai (West India), 13.5% in Chennai (South India), 16.6% in Hyderabad (South India), 12.4 % in Bangalore (South India) (Ramachandran et al., 2007). In *The National Urban Diabetes Survey* (*NUDS*), a population-based study was conducted in six metropolitan (Delhi, Mumbai, Kolkata, Chennai, Hyderabad, Bangalore) cities across India and recruited 11,216 subjects aged 20 years and above, representative of all socio-economic strata (Ramachandran et al., 2001). This study reported the age-standardized prevalence of type 2 diabetes as 12.1 per cent. Another study conducted in western India showed age-standardized prevalence of 8.6 per cent in urban population (Gupta et al., 2003). The Amrita Diabetes and Endocrine Population Survey (ADEPS), a community-based cross-sectional survey done in urban areas of Ernakulum district in Kerala have revealed a very high prevalence of 19.5 per cent (Menon et al., 2006).

Undiagnosed diabetes is also the hidden danger for India. Although studies for prevalence have clearly reflected the rate of diabetes among the Indian population but also have reported the very high prevalence of undiagnosed diabetes. Chennai Urban

Rural Epidemiology Study (CURES) established the undiagnosed-prevalence rate of 9.1% (Mohan et al., 2006). Similarly, Amrita Diabetes and Endocrine Population Survey (ADEPS) showed a prevalence rate of diagnosed and undiagnosed as 9.0% and 10.5% respectively (Menon et al., 2006). Kashmir Valley has undiagnosed diabetes prevalence rate of 4.25% (Zargar et al., 2000). The difference in urban and rural prevalence rate of diabetes was reported by the study of ICMR as 2.1% and 1.5% respectively (Ahuja et al., 1979). A later study showed a prevalence rate of urban (8.2%) and rural (2.4%) (Ramachandran et al., 2007). A study on the prevalence of diabetes in India study (PODIS) also reported the prevalence rate of diabetes in urban and rural population as 4.7% and 2.0 % respectively according to American Diabetes Association (ADA) criteria (Sadikot et al., 2004) and 5.6% and 2.7% respectively according to World Health Organization (WHO) criteria (Sadikot et al., 2004; Mohan et al., 2007). The individuals who are undiagnosed for DM and left untreated are more prone to micro-vascular and macro-vascular complications. Thus, it is strictly necessary to diagnose the precise and accurate prevalence rate of DM in Indian population.

2.2. Forms of Diabetes:

2.2.1. Type 1 diabetes:

T1DM is the result of severe insulin deficiency leading to insulin dependent DM. Though more frequently seen in those who develop diabetes during childhood or young adulthood, it can also occur at a later stage. In developed countries, almost all patients have the immune-mediated form of the disease. It is an auto-immune disease in which antibodies are produced thereby destroying the insulin-producing cells of the pancreas (Noble et al., 2012). Though unclear causes prevail, it is believed that both genetic and environmental factors may be involved. Idiopathic diabetes where no cause can be found is extremely rare. Type 1 diabetes is the second most cause of chronic disease after asthma. The highest incidence of type 1 A (autoimmune) diabetes is in Finland and the island of Sardinia (Songini et al., 2010). The frequency of type 1A diabetes is higher in Europe with rest of the world, higher in temperate zones and developed countries, co-relating with gross national product as an index of wealth. Type 1 B (idiopathic) diabetes has been noted in Japanese patients who progress rapidly to insulin dependence in adult life without diabetes associated anti-bodies but with increased serum amylase consistent with sub-acute pancreatitis (Urakami et al., 2012). The incidence of T1DM is increasing particularly under the age of 5 years. In a multicentre study, based on 2002-2003 data, 15,000 young people in the United States of America (USA) have newly diagnosed with T1DM annually (Dabelea et al., 2007).

2.2.2. Type 2 Diabetes:

T2DM is a common chronic disease of global importance. Most patients with (>85%) with diabetes have type 2 diabetes. The rate of increase of T2DM is such that there is effectively a global epidemic of it. T2DM is generally viewed as a clinical syndrome with variable phenotypic expressions (β- cells insufficiency and insulin resistance), however in most instances, the exact cause seems to be polygenic in nature and yet not known. The complexity of the pathogenesis of T2DM reflects the heterogeneous genetic, pathologic, environmental and metabolic abnormalities that exist in the different patients, but the ultimate expression of the hyperglycemic state involves some combination of impaired insulin secretion from the β-cells of pancreas, insulin resistance and increased glucose production from the liver. This form encompasses to those who have insulin resistance and usually have a relative (rather than absolute) deficiency of insulin. People with this diabetes form are insulin resistant (DeFronzo et al., 1997 and Lillioja et al., 1993). Type 2 diabetes is frequently undiagnosed for a long time because of the insincerity of hyperglycemia in the body that shows the symptoms (Mooy et al., 1995 and Harris et al., 1993). The majority of patients with this form of diabetes mellitus are obese thereby causing insulin resistance (Campbell et al., 1993 and Bogardus et al., 1985). Those patients who are not obese may represent fat deposition in abdominal region changing into central obesity (Kissebah et al., 1982). Ketoacidosis in association with infections is frequently associated with this form of diabetes (Banerji et al., 1994 and Umpierrez et al., 1995). Diabetes has been traditionally considered as a disease of economically rich countries. However, recent data suggests that 80% of people with diabetes live in countries classified by the World Bank as low- and middle-income countries, and this proportion is set to increase. The prevalence of T2DM is related to increasing age, increasing calorie intake, increasing obesity and reducing physical activity. Pregnancy, certain drug therapy, and inter-current illness are well associated with precipitating diabetes. In all patients with T2DM, there is both insulin resistance and relative insulin deficiency.

2.2.3. Maturity Onset Diabetes of Young (MODY):

MODY is a rare form of a heterogeneous group of disorders resulting in beta cell dysfunction. It is distinct from insulin dependent and non-insulin dependent diabetes. These are unified by being forms of DM with a strong family history and early onset, usually in children or adolescents. The clinical hallmark of MODY is a mild increased in blood sugar in child, adolescent or young with strong family history of diabetes (Reinehr et al., 2013). The current estimates suggest that MODY accounts for 1 to 5% of all diabetes cases in USA and other westernized countries (Murea et al., 2012). MODY is considered as a group of diabetic condition distinctive from type 1 and type 2 diabetes. MODY is inherited in auto-somal dominant way with numerous forms.

The genetic basis of MODY indicates that genetic mutations result in diabetes by primarily effecting β-cell functions (Yamagata et al., 1996). MODY is also referred to as "monogenic diabetes" (Edghill et al., 2006). MODY results from mutation in genes such as, GCK (glycolytic enzyme glucokinase), HNF-4-α (hepatocyte nuclear factor 4-α), HNF1A (hepatocye nuclear factor 1- α), PDX1 (pancreatic/duodenum homeobox protein-1), HNF1B (hepatocye nuclear factor 1-β) and NEUROD1 (neurogenic differentiation factor-1). In the main, they do not present ketosis and weight loss as in T1DM, and there is no strong connection with obesity as for T2DM.

2.2.4. Gestational diabetes mellitus (GDM):

GDM develops when a typical glucose tolerance develops during pregnancy in a woman not known to have diabetes before pregnancy. The women with GDM are quite likely to develop it again in a subsequent pregnancy and are at considerably increased risk of developing type 2 diabetes in future (Wendland et al., 2012). Although most of the cases of this form of diabetes resolve with delivery. After deliberations in 2008-2009, the International Association of Diabetes and Pregnancy Study Groups (IADPSG) including American Diabetes Association (ADA) recommended that high-risk women found to have diabetes mellitus at their prenatal visit with standard diagnostic criteria, receive a diagnosis of overt, not gestational diabetes. Nearly 7% pregnancies are complicated with GDM (Hearth et al., 2017).

The statistical figure reflects that about 1.5-2.5 times more insulin is secreted than in normal pregnancy (Carr and Gabbe, 1998). Glucose travels freely through facilitated diffusion by GLUT1 located in the syncytiotrophoblast on basal membranes. If the GDM is untreated, the fetus is exposed to hyperglycemia that leads to fetal insulin at a high level leading to excessive growth and macrosomia. The precise mechanism underlying the causes of gestational diabetes is unknown. Insulin resistance may be the probable cause for GDM, as pregnancy hormones (placental) along with other unknown (fat depositions) factors binds with insulin receptors causing insulin resistance (Carr and Gabbe, 1998). The risk factors for GDM includes older age, obesity, history of poor pregnancy outcome, a history of large for gestational age babies, and belonging to a racial/ ethnic group with a known high occurrence of type 2 diabetes (ADA., 2003).

2.2.5. Neonatal diabetes:

Neonatal diabetes develops in neonate shortly after the birth and within 2 years of life. It can be transient or permanent (Aguilar-Bryan et al., 2008). It is due to defect in potassium channel of insulin secreting cells, as a result of mutations in genes which limit the closure of potassium channels and therefore insulin secretion (Ashcroft et al., 2005). The gene mutation can be rectified by sulphonylureas which enables the activation of potassium channel (Hattersley et al., 2005).

2.3. Diagnostic Criteria:

DM is characterized by increased blood glucose concentrations which can vary as a continuum in different people.

Table 2: Criteria for diagnosis of DM according to ADA Guidelines (ADA, 2014)

➢ **Fasting plasma glucose ≥126 mg/dL (7.0 mmol/L)* (Fasting is defined as no caloric intake for atleast ≥8 hours*)**/ OR
➢ **2-hr post prandial glucose ≥200 mg/dL (11.1 mmol/L) during oral glucose tolerance test. The test should be performed as described by WHO using a glucose load containing the equivalent of 75 gm anhydrous glucose dissolved in water** (OR) **(Using a glucose load containing the equivalent of 75g anhydrous glucose dissolved in water*)**
➢ **A1C ≥6.5% (48 mmol/mol)**/OR
➢ **In a patient with classic symptoms of hyperglycemia or hyperglycemic crisis, in random plasma glucose ≥200 mg/dL (11.1 mmol/L).**

2.4. Pathogenesis:

2.4.1. Pathogenesis of Type 1 Diabetes Mellitus:

T1DM is defined as a chronic autoimmune disorder associated with selective insulin-producing pancreatic β-cells destruction (Atkinson et al., 2012). It is characterized by the presence of islet cell specific autoantibodies, immunocompetent and accessory cells in infiltrated pancreatic islets, altered T-cell mediated autoregulation and a susceptibility to disease with the class II genes of the major histo-compatibility complex (MHC); human leukocyte antigens (HLA) (Bottazo et al., 1974). In addition to the declined insulin secretion, the function of pancreatic α-cells is also abnormal, and there is unnecessary secretion of glucagon in patients (Bottazo et al., 1985). After effects of insulin deficiency lead to uncontrolled lipolysis and high levels of free fatty acids in plasma, which deforms glucose metabolism in peripheral tissue, thus impairing glucose consumption. Insulin deficiency also hinders the expression of some genes necessary for target tissues to respond normally to insulin via the GLUT 4, class of glucose transporters in adipose tissue and glucokinase in liver (Lin et al., 2011). The major metabolic derangements, which result from insulin deficiency in insulin-dependent diabetes mellitus (IDDM), are impaired glucose, lipid and protein metabolism. Under normal physiological situation, plasma glucose levels are maintained within a narrow range, despite wide fluctuations in demand and supply, through a tightly regulated and dynamic relation between insulin sensitivity and tissue sensitivity to insulin (especially in liver).

The aetiology of type 1 diabetes is unknown but like other complex diseases, the outcome of T1DM is determined by the interplay of multiple genes and (most likely) multiple environmental determinants, together with an element of happenstance (Gillispie et al., 2006). Relative insulin deficiency is found in both types of diabetes, but marked insulin deficiency with normal or near-normal insulin sensitivity is the hallmark of type 1 diabetes. Even low rates of insulin secretion are sufficient to inhibit ketogenesis in the liver, which is why diabetic ketoacidosis is characteristic of type 1 but not type 2 diabetes. Prospective studies of children at high risk of type 1 diabetes have shown that beta cell function declines over many months or years before clinical onset (Faideu et al., 2005). Autoimmune processes undoubtedly mediate many pathological consequences of T1DM (Atiknson et al., 2015). Evidence for this includes the overlap between type 1 diabetes and other HLA-associated autoimmmune conditions, the presence of insulitis (lymphocytic infiltration of the islets) in newly diagnosed children, evidence of humoral and cellular immunity directed against islet constituents, the observation of passive transfer of diabetes from marrow donors to recipients, the re-enactment of autoimmunity in twin-to-twin transplants, and the response to immunosuppressive therapy in the newly diagnosed.

2.4.2. Pathogenesis of Type 2 Diabetes Mellitus:

The pathogenesis of T2DM is complex and involves the interaction of environmental and genetic factors. The excessive calorie intake and sedentary lifestyle are environmental causes playing a crucial in role in causing T2DM. In T2DM, two main pathological defects occurs a) impaired insulin secretion through a pancreatic β-cell dysfunction, and impaired insulin action via insulin resistance (Holt., 2004). β-cell failure occurs much earlier and is more severe. Subjects in the upper limit of impaired glucose tolerance (IGT) are maximally/near maximally insulin resistant and have lost about 80% of their β-cell functioning. In addition to the muscle, liver, and β-cell (triumvirate), accelerated lipolysis, incretin deficiency/resistance, hyperglucagonemia, increased glucose reabsorption, and role of central nervous system in metabolic regulation, all play important roles in the development of glucose intolerance in type 2 diabetic individuals (Defronzo et al., 1992) (Figure 2). Although the precise way in which genetic, environmental and patho-physiological factors interact to lead to the clinical onset of T2DM is not known, understanding of these processes has increased substantially. With the exception to some monogenic form of disease that might result from defects largely confined to pathways that regulate insulin action in muscle, liver and fat or defects in insulin secretory functions in pancreatic beta cell, it is currently believed that the common forms of T2DM are polygenic in nature and are caused by combination of insulin resistance, abnormal insulin secretion, and other factors (Tallapragada et al., 2015). From patho-physiological point of view, it is the inability of the pancreatic beta cell to adapt to the reductions in insulin sensitivity that occurs over a lifetime that precipitates the onset of T2DM. The most common factors that place an increased secretory burden on the beta cell are puberty, pregnancy, a sedentary lifestyle, and overeating leading to weight gain. An underlying genetic predisposition appears to be critical factor in determining the frequency with which beta cell failure occur (Halban et al., 2014). Individuals with T2DM have detectable levels of circulating insulin, unlike patients with type 1 diabetes. Subjects with impaired glucose tolerance have a hyperglycemic state in spite of evident plasma insulin level, indicating their resistance to insulin action. Therefore progression from insulin resistance to the development of type 2 diabetes, insulin level tapers down indicating type 2 diabetic have less insulin secretion

2.4.2.1. __Defective Insulin Secretion and Processing__

Type 2 diabetes is characterized by diminished or inappropriate secretion of insulin, which could be a defect of either islet cell function or -cell mass (Clark et al., 2001). Type 2 diabetes is a multi-factorial disorder, secondary to a reduction in glucose uptake and excessive liver glucose production, associated with a joint decrease in insulin secretion and insulin sensitivity (Guillausseau et al., 2008). Slight changes in the dynamics of insulin secretion exists which may have significant effects on insulin action and efficiency. In normal subjects, a hasty rise in glucose levels induces a a two phase insulin response. The first phase is rapid in onset and temporary, lasting about 5-10 minutes. However, the second phase occurs more slowly and lasts for the duration of the hyperglycaemia. Although most of the insulin is secreted during the second phase insulin response, the first phase is a more competent signal, serving an vital physiological role to maximize glucose clearance and 'prime' the liver to close down glucose synthesis (Leahy et al., 1992). In type 2 diabetes, the first phase insulin response is dull and accounts in part for the exaggerated post-prandial rise in plasma glucose evident in these subjects. In established disease the second phase insulin response is also weakened and at this stage it is unclear whether defects in first or second phase insulin secretion have a larger impact on glycaemia. Once hyperglycemia is established, insulin secretion declines with time due to glucotoxicity and lipotoxicity (Guillausseau et al., 2008).

*2.4.2.2. **<u>Insulin Resistance</u>***

Insulin resistance is define as an impaired biological response to endogenously produce insulin or exogenously administered insulin in the body. The disorders in metabolism of amino-acids, glucose and lipids are present in insulin resistant individual (Wilcox et al., 2005). Insulin resistance, by placing an increased demand on the β-cell to hypersecrete insulin, also plays an important role in the progressive β-cell failure of type 2 diabetes. Insulin resistance plays a central role in development of impaired glucose tolerance and diabetes mellitus. Prospective studies have suggested that insulin resistance predicts the onset of diabetes mellitus. During insulin resistance there is a failure in stimulation of glucose uptake in peripheral tissues and suppression in hepatic glucose output (Garvey., 1992).

Insulin resistance involves both muscle and liver. In the basal state, the liver represents a major location of insulin resistance, and this is reflected by over synthesis of hepatic glucose despite the presence of fasting hyperinsulinemia and hyperglycemia. This accelerated rate of hepatic glucose output is the key determinant of the elevated fasting plasma glucose concentration in type 2 diabetic individuals. In type 2 diabetic individuals, the rate of basal hepatic glucose production is increased, averaging -2.5 mg/kg per min (Defronzo et al., 1992).

Muscle insulin resistance could account for over 85–90% of the impairment in total body glucose disposal in type 2 diabetic subjects (Pedengrass et al., 2007). Although glucose uptake by muscle glucose in the postabsorptive state is increased when viewed in absolute terms, the efficiency of the glucose clearance is reduced. After glucose infusion or ingestion (i.e., in the insulin stimulated state) both decreased muscle glucose uptake and impaired suppression of HGP contribute to the insulin resistance. Other sites of insulin resistance include adipocytes and the liver. An incapability of insulin to restrain lipolysis in adipocytes results in increased plasma levels of non-esterified fatty acids (NEFA) that triggers gluconeogenesis, triglyceride synthesis and glucose production in the liver. They also reduce glucose uptake and utilisation by skeletal muscle and decrease the extraction of insulin from portal blood by the liver (Chatterjee et al., 2002). However, under euglycemic hyperinsulinemic conditions, HPG is largely suppressed and impaired muscle glucose uptake is primarily responsible for the insulin resistance. There are numerous causes and determinants of insulin resistance. There is evidence that insulin resistance is transmitted as a polygenic familial trait in some populations, e.g. the Pima Indians, although the genes liable are largely unexplored (Chatterjee et al., 2002).

2.4.4.3. ***Role of obesity***

Obesity is strongly associated with type 2 diabetes (Yajnik et al., 2009). The Pima Indians have a very high incidence of obesity and have the highest prevalence of diabetes in the world (Krosnick ., 2000). A number of large prospective studies have evaluated the association of risk of diabetes and development of insulin resistance with increase in body fat content (Patel et al., 2013). A BMI of >35 kg/m2 predicts a 40-fold greater risk of disease development compared to a BMI of < 25 kg/m^2. Central distribution of adipose tissue is particularly more strongly associated with insulin resistance to also with other variables such as TAGs concentration, total plasma cholesterol, decreased HDL concentration (Paniagua., 2016). In this context visceral versus subcutaneous fat thickness has more pathogenic importance, attributable perhaps to increased production of NEFA (reaching the liver directly through the portal system. nterestingly, truncal obesity has been correlated with an increased proportion of fast twitch (white) to red fibres in skeletal muscle with low levels of insulin binding and decreased insulin sensitivity. Truncal obesity is partly inherited but also associated with a sedentary life style (Chatterjee et al. 2002). Putative obesity genes include those encoding metabolic enzymes that could lead to insulin resistance in skeletal muscle e.g. glycogen synthetase, insulin receptor substrate 1, or those that interfere with normal homeostatic control of the fat mass, e.g. β3 adrenoreceptor, leptin receptor. By predisposing to fat storage, such genes may confer the ‘thrifty genotype’, which in times of famine represented a survival advantage but in modern society results in obesity and type 2 diabetes (Joffe et al., 1998).

*2.4.4.4. **Islet amyloid***

Islet amyloid are made up of insoluble fibrils formed from IAPP (co-secreted with insulin) may also play a role in type 2 diabetes pathogenesis. Islet amyloid progressively replaces the β-cell mass and the degree of islet replacement influences therapy: patients with extensive amyloidosis typically require insulin, implying that amyloid deposition impairs islet function, which may be important in the decline in insulin secretion in the later stages of the disease (De Fronzo et al., 2002). The aetiology of amyloid formation is unknown but it has been suggested that an alteration in β-cell function related to increased dietary fat intake results in a change in production, processing and/or secretion of IAPP, critical to the initial formation of islet amyloid fibrils (Kahn et al., 1999).

*2.4.4.5. **Glucose toxicity***

The most possible elucidation for an acquired defective insulin secretion relates to the notion of glucose toxicity – that is, hindered β-cell responsiveness to a glucose stimulus in the face of hyperglycemia, so that small increases in glucose concentration in this state do not evoke appropriate rise in insulin synthesis (Chatterjee et al., 2002). This does not necessarily infer toxicity on the β-cell per se as it is already operating at a higher level along the stimulus–response curve. Moreover, in a rat model of diabetes induced by partial pancreatectomy, hyperglycaemia has been associated with impaired insulin secretion but normo-glycaemia induced by phlorizin (a renal tubular poison increasing urinary glucose loss without a direct effect on the β-cell) restored a normal insulin response, suggesting a reversible effect of hyperglycaemia on β-cells. In humans, evidence is equivocal, but the observation that good glycaemic control increases β-cell function supports the hypothesis that hyperglycaemia has an adverse effect on insulin secretion (DeFronzo et al., 1992).

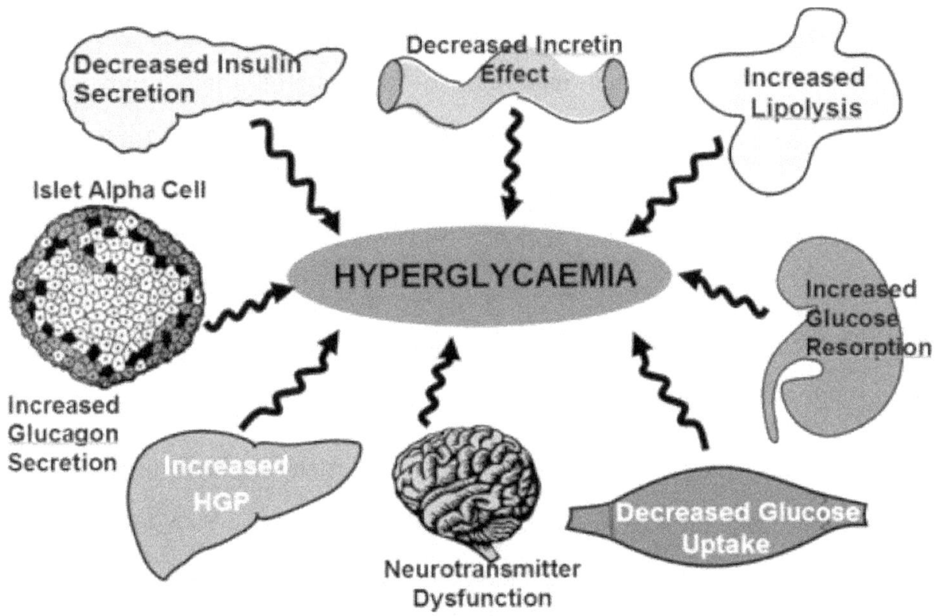

Figure 2: The omnious octet and pathogenesis of type 2 diabetes (Adapted from DeFronzo et al., 1992).

2.4.3. Mechanism of Hyperglycemia Mediated Damage:

The diabetic complications are caused by prolonged exposure to high glucose levels; the extent of diabetic tissue damage is also determined by genetic determinants of individual susceptibility independent accelerating factors as such as hypertension and dyslipidemia. The murine animal models are important tools for defining the pathogenesis of diabetes associated complications. But few limitations associated with such diabetic model recapitulate the structural and functional alterations of human complications. For eg. Rodents do not develop proliferative retinopathy, coronary atherosclerosis and interstitial fibrosis. The dominant mechanisms involved differ at different stages of diabetic complications. The molecular mechansism needs to be explored in each complication associated target tissue. In addition, only 33-50% of subjects with diabetes poor glycemic control will develop nephropathy, and a subset of patients with good glycemic control still develops nephropathy. Since rodent models do not develop progressive complications resembling human diabetic, without analysis from human tissues, exploration of possible protective factors preventing subjects with poor glycemic control to develop ESRD is not possible. By using primary human cell lines and mouse models for major hypothesis regarding hyperglycemia induced diabetic complications have generated a large amount of data as well as several clinical trials based on specific inhibitors of mechanisms. The role of hyperglycemia has been established by large-scale prospective studies for both type 1 and type 2 diabetes, the Diabetes Control and Complications Trial (DCCT., 1993) and the UK Prospective Diabetes Study (UKPDS., 1996). Similar results have also been reported by Steno study (Gaede et al., 2008).

There are four major hypotheses leading to diabetic complications including increased intracellular formation of advanced glycation end products (AGEs), increased polyol pathway flux, activation of protein kinase-C pathway and increased hexosamine pathway flux.

2.4.3.1. <u>Advanced Glycation End product Formation</u>:

AGEs originally arise from non-enzymatic glycation between extracellular and intracellular proteins and glucose. One theory is that due to chronic hyperglycemia in diabetes there is accelerated non-enzymatic glycation resulting in formation of AGEs by the so-called Maillard reaction (Maillard., 1912). In normal individuals, glucose reacts with the amine group of proteins to form some amount of early glycated products (Amadori glucose) through the non-enzymatic and irreversible process. It has also arisen from intra-cellular auto-oxidation of glucose to glyoxal, decomposition of amadori product to 3-deoxygluconase, and fragmentation of glyceraldehydes-3-phosphate to methylglyoxal (Brownlee et al., 2001). These reactive intracellular dicarbonyl reacts with amino groups of intracellular and extracellular proteins to form AGEs. There are various mechanisms explain the damage of target cells caused by intracellular production of AGEs precursor. AGEs acts as recognition signals for uptake and degradation of proteins by macrophages resulting in the production of cytokines, and growth factors such like tumor necrosis factor α (TNF-α), Interleukin 1 (IL-1), insulin like growth factor 1 (IGF-1), granulocyte-macrophage colony-stimulating factor (GM-CSF) and platelet-derived growth factor (PDGF) and inducing receptor-mediated reactive oxygen species (ROS) production. Modification of matrix proteins such as type 1 collagen, type 4 collagen, and laminins also occurs resulting in change in structure and function of extracellular matrix most importantly reduction in endothelial cell adhesion. AGE-modified proteins can also alter cellular function through binding to specific AGE receptor (RAGE) on endothelial cells. RAGE belongs to a class of immunoglobulin superfamily is expressed on the surface of a variety of cell types, including endothelial cells, smooth muscle cells, lymphocytes, monocytes, and neurons. Activation of RAGE triggers the generation of reactive oxygen species and further activation of signaling molecules such as nuclear factor Kb, p21, and protein kinase C (PKC) (Brownlee et al., 2001) (Figure 3).

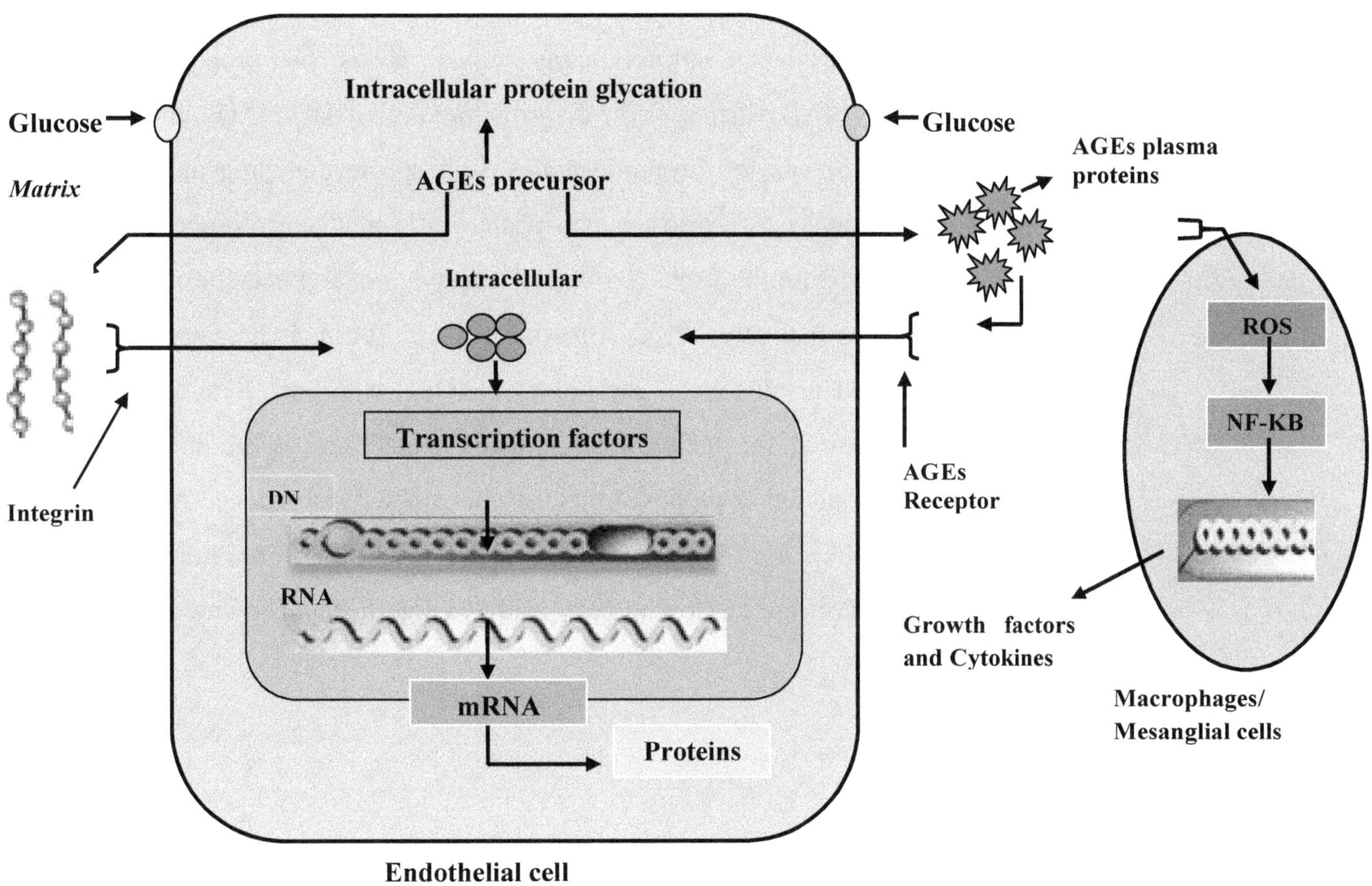

Figure 3: Increased production of AGE precursors and its pathologic consequences. (Adapted from Brownlee M: Biochemistry and molecular cell biology of diabetic complications. Nature 414:813–820, 2001).

*2.4.3.2. **Polyol Pathway Flux:***

Normally intracellular glucose is predominantly phosphorylated to glucose-6-phosphate by the enzyme hexokinase to be metabolized later on by glycolysis and hexosamine mono-phosphate shunt (HMP), and only small amount is converted to sorbitol by the polyol pathway. Enzyme aldose reductase is the rate-limiting step in this alternate pathway, and it has low affinity for glucose (Brownlee et al., 2001). Under hyperglycemic conditions, there is increased the flux of glucose through this pathway that is about 30% and is metabolized this way. In a hyperglycemic environment, however, increased intracellular glucose results in increased enzymatic conversion to the polyalcohol sorbitol, with a concomitant decrease in nicotinamide adenine dinucleotide phosphate (NADPH). The mechanism by which glucose flux through the polyol is detrimental and not clearly defined. It has been proposed that oxidation of sorbitol by NAD+ increases the cytosolic ratio of NADH/NAD+, thereby inhibiting the activity of enzyme glyceraldehydes 3-phosphate dehydrogenase and increasing concentrations of triose phosphate. Elevated triose-phosphate concentrations could increase the formation of both methylglyoxal precursor of AGE and diacylglycerol, thus activating PKC (Brownlee et al., 2001). It has also been found that the reduction of glucose to sorbitol by NADPH consumes the co-factor NADPH which is required for regenerating reduced glutathione is an important cellular anti-oxidant. Some other proposed mechanisms are sorbitol-induced osmotic stress and decreased NA+, K+ ATPase activity. But the sorbitol concentration in diabetic vessels and nerves are too low to be considered significant (Brownlee et al., 2003) (Figure 4).

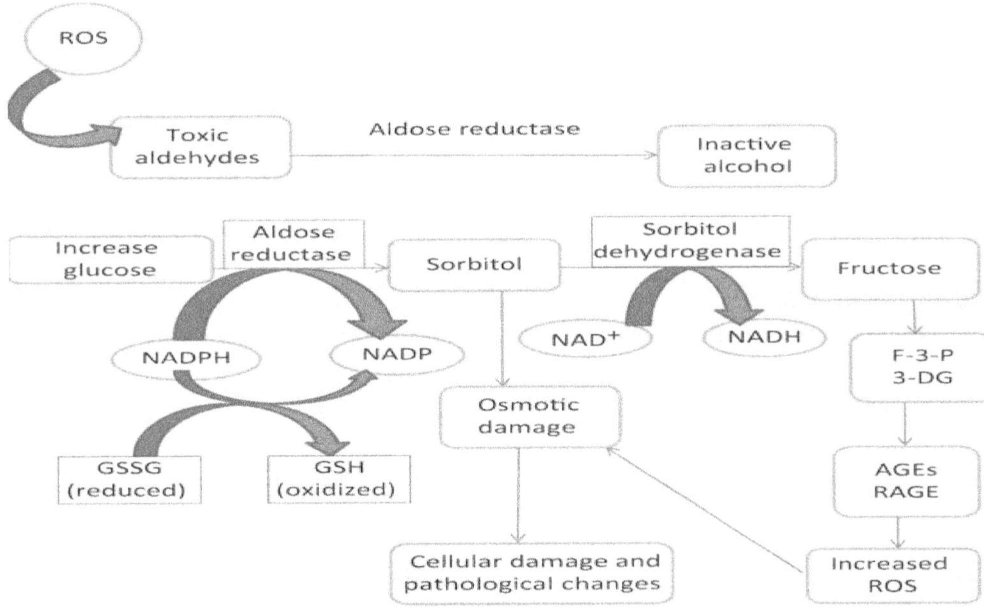

Figure 4: Hyperglycemia increases flux through the hexosamine pathway. (Adapted from Brownlee M: Biochemistry and molecular cell biology of diabetic complications. Nature 414:813–820, 2001).

2.4.3.3. Activation of Protein Kinase C (PKC):

The third important mechanism is the activation of family of PKC enzymes which are cell signaling enzymes. These enzymes are involved in the cellular functions ranging from cell growth and differentiation, apoptosis, protein trafficking, cytoskeletal rearrangement and cell polarity. PKC forms area activated by second messenger diacylglycerol (DAG). In states of hyperglycemia, there is increased concentration of DAG as a result of its de-novo synthesis from glyceraldehydes-3-phosphate.). In a study conducted on diabetic rats, it was found that increased DAG content primarily activates the PKC β and δ isoforms along with PKC-α and PKC-ε in the retina (Koya et al., 1998) and PKC-α and δ in the glomerulus (Koya et al., 1997). An abnormal pattern of PKC pathway in diabetes mellitus has shown to be involved in decreased glomerular and smooth muscle cells NO production (Craven et al., 1994). PKC activation in hyperglycemic conditions inhibits insulin-stimulated expression of eNOS messenger RNA (mRNA) in cultured endothelial cells (Pugliese et al., 1994). Activation of PKC has been associated with suppression of nitric oxide production via inhibition of insulin-stimulated expression of endothelial nitric oxide synthase (eNOS) and stimulation of endothelin 1 (ET-10) vasoconstrictor activity. It also leads to increased microvascular matrix protein accumulation by inducing the expression of tumor growth factor beta-1 (TGF-β1), fibronectin, and type IV collagen. It has also been implicated in the overexpression of the fibrinolytic inhibitor PAI-1 and the activation of pleiotropic transcription factor NF-Kb. It also induces expression of the permeability-enhancing factor vascular endothelial growth factor (VEGF) (Brownlee et al., 2001) (Figure 5).

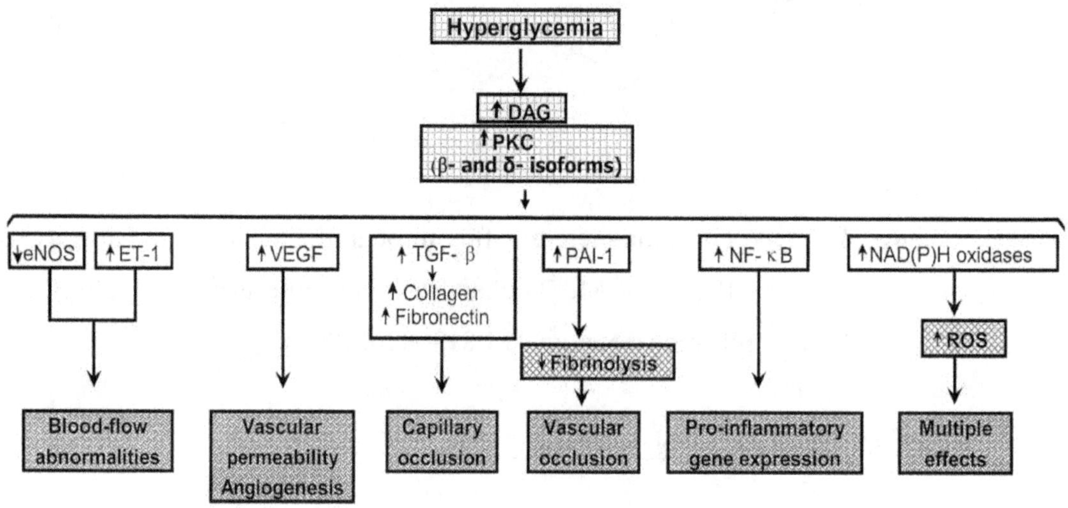

Figure 5: Potential consequences of hyperglycemia-induced PKC activation. (Adapted from Williams textbook of Endocrinology 11th Ed)

2.4.3.4. __Hexosamine pathway:__

The fourth hypothesis is that in states of hyperglycemia there is a flux of glucose through hexosamine pathway. In this pathway, fructose-6-phosphate leaving from glycolysis acts as a substrate for the reactions that require uridine diphosphate-N-acetylglucosamine (UDP-GlcNAc) in O-linked glycoprotein synthesis. It is one of the normal sugar metabolic mechanism occurs in various tissues that encounter less amount of glucose. The increased glucose flux through hexosamine pathway mediates hyperglycemia-induced activation of Sp1 sites that regulate hyperglycemia – induced activation of the PAI-1 promoter in smooth muscle cells (Chen et al., 1998).

In a previous study, it has been found that there is an increase of 2.4 fold in hexosamine pathway activity in endothelial cells that result in 1.7 fold increases in Sp1-O-linked GlcNAc and a 70% to 80% decrease in Sp1 O-linked phosphothreonine and phosphoserine (Du et al., 2001). PAI-1 promoter regulation requires PKC-β1 and PKC-δ in hexosamine pathway in endothelial cells (Goldberg et al., 2002). In another study, GlcNAc modification of Sp1 also regulates glucose-responsive expression of the pro sclerotic growth factor TGF-β1. ROS production inhibits GAPDH resulting in accumulation of oxidized metabolites like leading to over-activation of hexosamine cascade (Brownlee et al., 2001) (Figure 6).

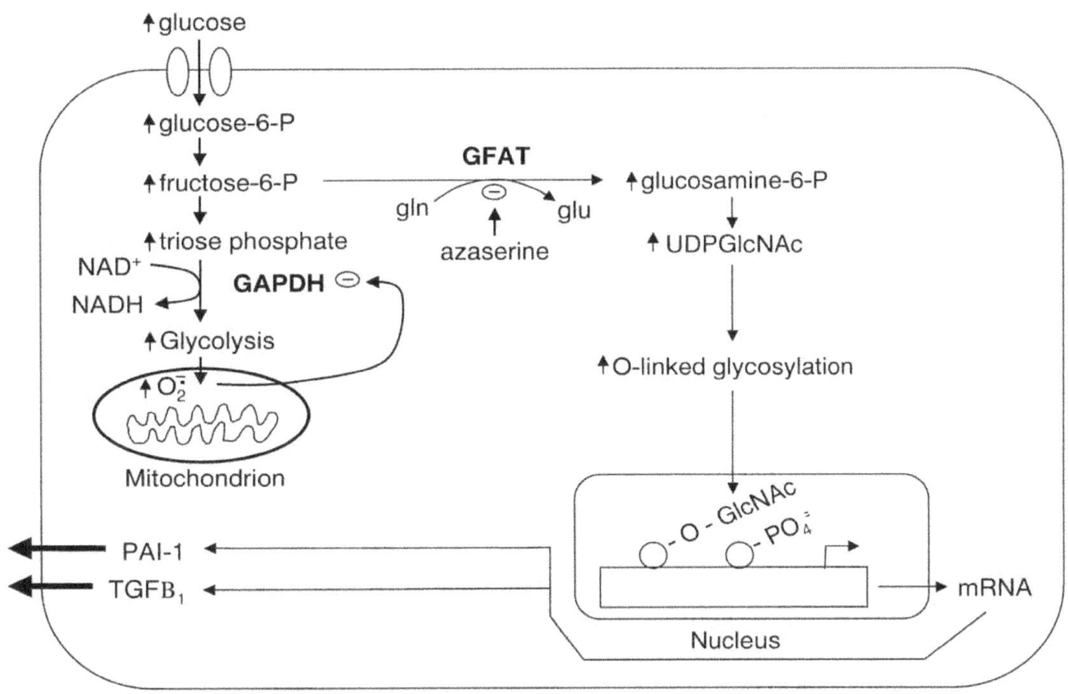

Figure 6: Schematic representation of hexosamine pathway. (Adapted from Williams textbook of Endocrinology 11th Ed.)

2.4.3.5 <u>Reactive Oxygen species and Hyperglycemia</u>:

ROS are formed from the reduction of molecular oxygen or by oxidation of water to yield superoxide anion, hydrogen peroxide, nitric oxide and hydroxyl radicals. Mitochondria and NADPH oxidases are major sources of ROS production. Hyperglycemia enhances the oxidation of glucose in the mitochondria, further, resulting in increase voltage across electron tansport chain in inner mitochondrial membrane. Increase in voltage is due to shuttling down of electrons between the complexes I, II and III from the increase in reducing equivalents NADH and FADH synthesis from oxidation of intracellular excess glucose (Rolo et al., 2006). Ubiquinone transfers the electrons through the complexes I and II to complex III, cytochrome C, complex IV and finally to molecular oxygen (Wallace., 1999). The passage of electrons through the complexes leaks protons into the intra-mitochondrial space resulting in increased voltage, which in turn results in mitochondrial superoxide production (Logan., 2006). Normally, inactive poly ADP-ribose polymerase (PARP) enzyme resides in nucleus. PARP is responsible for making polymers of ADP-ribose. Superoxide activates PARP enzyme (Brownlee., 2005) and inhibits GAPDH (Brownlee., 2005; Nishikawa et al., 2000) (Figure 7).

GADPH is a cytosolic glycolytic pathway enzyme and catalysis glyceraldehydes-3-phosphate and dihydroxyacetone phosphate (DHAP) to glyceraldehydes-1,3-bisphosphate. Nicotianamide adnine dinucleotide is a co-factor and gets reduced to NADH during the reaction carried by GADPH. Activated PARP enzyme splits NAD+ into nicotinic acide and ADP-ribose (Kim et al., 2005), thus inhibiting formation of NADH (Brownlee., 2005; Giacco et al., 2010). Glycolytic substrates including glyceraldehydes-3-phosphate, fructose -6-phosphate, glucose-6-phosphate, and glucose gets accumulated leading to different pathways responsible for diabetic complications (Brownlee., 2005; Giacco et al., 2010).

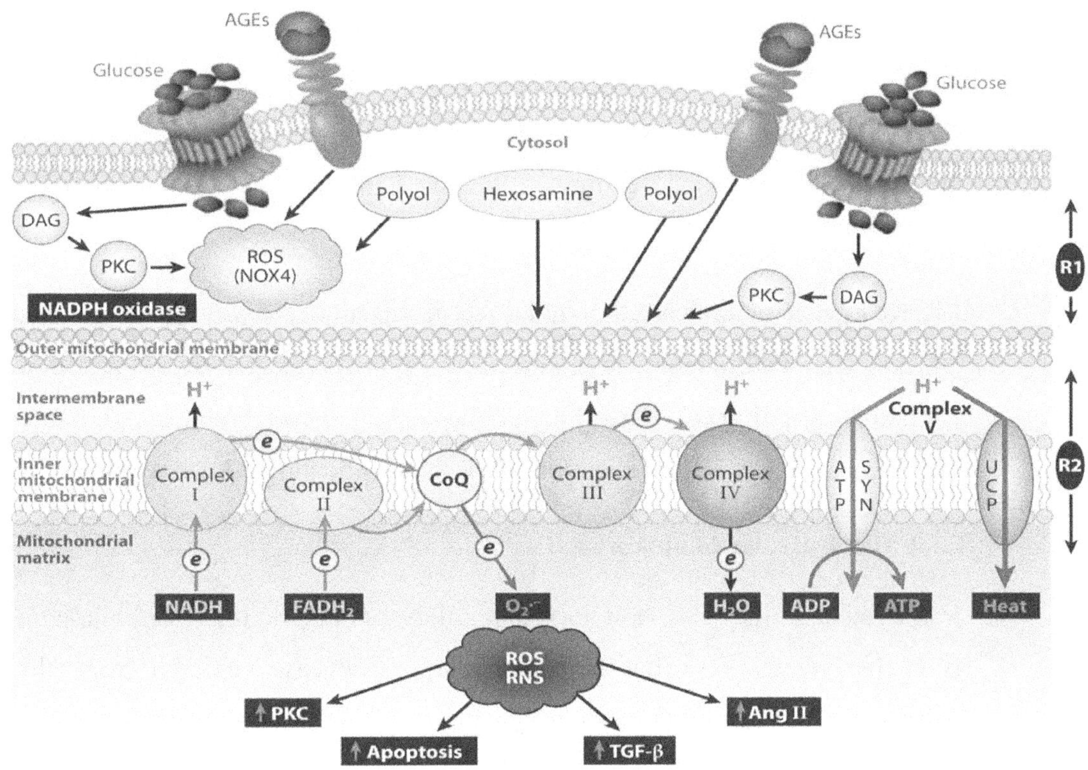

Figure 7: Production of ROS by the mitochondrial electron transport chain. (Adapted from Brownlee., 2005)

2. 5. Complications of Diabetes Mellitus:

Complications due to diabetes are a major cause of disability, morbidity, reduced quality of life, and mortality. Diabetes complications can affect different parts of the body manifesting in unusual ways for different people. Diabetes increases patients' risk for many serious health problems. In men, it is responsible for erectile dysfunction, low testosterone levels. According to ADA statistical analysis; heart disease is the leading cause of death in women with diabetes (ADA, 2005). In addition, women with DM are afflicted by depression, prone to sexual health problems and also eating disorders tend to occur more frequently.

Diabetes complications are divided into microvascular (due to damage to small blood vessels) and macrovascular (due to damage to larger blood vessels). Micro-vascular complications involve damage to eyes (retinopathy) leading to blindness, kidneys (nephropathy) causing renal failure and nerves (neuropathy) leading to impotence and diabetic foot disorders (which include severe infections and ultimately amputation). Foot complications can get worse in association with serious complications, such as neuropathy, skin changes, calluses as well as foot ulcers, and poor circulation (Aalto., 1997).

Macrovascular complications include cardiovascular diseases such as strokes, heart attacks, and insufficiency in blood flow to lower extremities. Various evidences explain the requirement of good metabolic control in both type 1 and 2 diabetes which can delay the onset and progression of these complications (Nyenwe et al., 2011).

2.5.1 Microvascular complications:

In the retina, kidney and vasa nervosum, diabetes-specific microvascular complication is characterized by similar pathophysiologic features. Research from clinical and animal data suggests that chronic hyperglycemia is the prime factor that initiates all diabetic microvascular disease. In the Diabetes Control and Complications Trials (DCCT) on T1DM subjects whose intensive insulin therapy resulted in haemoglobin A1c (HbA1c) levels 2% lower than those receiving conventional insulin therapy had a 76% lower incidence of retinopathy, a 54% lower incidence of nephropathy and a 60% reduction in neuropathy (DCCT Trial 1993).

*2.5.1.1. **Diabetic Retinopathy:***

Diabetic retinopathy is a considered as the foremost cause of blindness and visual dysfunction. The risk of developing diabetic retinopathy in diabetes is dependent on both the duration and the severity of hyperglycemia (National Diabetes Data Group, 1995). It is a result of damage caused by small blood vessel to the back layer of the eye, the retina, leading to progressive vision loss and in more severe cases causes blindness. Most patients with type 1 diabetes develop signs of retinopathy within 20 years of clinical diagnosis (UKPDS., 1998). Confirmation of early changes in the blood vessels of the retina can be made through regular eye examinations. Diabetic retinopathy is usually classified as either background or proliferative retinopathy (Aiello et al., 1998). Background retinopathy includes features such as small hemorrhages in the middle layers of the retina. They are clinically seen as “dots” and therefore ,are commonly referred to as “dot hemorrhages.” Proliferative retinopathy is characterized by the formation of new blood vessels on the surface of the retina that may lead to vitreous hemorrhage. White areas on the retina (“cotton wool spots”) can be a sign of imminent proliferative retinopathy. Laser photocoagulation can often prevent proliferative retinopathy from progressing to blindness; therefore, close surveillance for the existence or progression of retinopathy in patients with diabetes is crucial (Monson et al., 1986).

2.5.1.2. __Diabetic Nephropathy__:

Diabetic kidney disease is also caused by damage to small blood vessels in the kidneys. This can cause kidney failure and eventually, lead to death. In developed countries, this is a leading cause of dialysis and kidney transplant. It is defined by proteinuria >500 mg in 24 h in the diabetic subjects, but this is preceded by microalbuminuria (Shihabi et al., 1991). Microalbuminuria is defined as albumin excretion of 30-299 mg/24 h. Diabetic nephropathy is the leading cause of ESKD in the United States and a leading cause of DM related morbidity and mortality. Both micro-albuminuria and macro-albuminuria in individuals with DM are associated with increased risk of cardio-vascular diseases (Weir et al., 2007). The pathological disturbances to the kidney include increased glomerular basement membrane thickness, microaneurysm formation, mesangial nodule formation (Kimmelsteil-Wilson bodies) (Alsaad et al., 2007). Hyperglycemia in DM causes abnormalities in blood flow and vascular permeability in the glomerulus. The increase in blood flow rate and intra-capillary pressure is thought to contribute hyperglycemia-induced declined nitric oxide (NO) on the efferent side of the capillary beds and possibly an increased production of angiotensin II, which results in the leakage of fluorescein and glomerular capillaries have elevated albumin excretion rate (AER). If diagnosed at an early stage, several measures can retard the progression to kidney failure. These include control of high blood glucose, control of high blood pressure, intervention with medication in the early stage of kidney damage, and restriction of dietary protein (Levin., 2008).

2.5.1.3. <u>Diabetic Neuropathy</u>:

Diabetic neuropathy is recognized by the ADA (ADA, 2007) as "the presence of symptoms and signs of peripheral nerve dysfunction in people with diabetes after the exclusion of other causes." As with other micro-vascular complications, the risk of developing diabetic neuropathy is proportional to both the magnitude and duration of hyperglycemia, and some individuals may possess genetic attributes that affect their predisposition to developing such complications. The precise nature of the injury to the peripheral nerves from hyperglycemia is not known but likely is related to mechanisms such as polyol accumulation, injury from AGEs, and oxidative stress. More than 80% of amputations occur after foot ulceration or injury, which can result from diabetic neuropathy. The diabetes control and complications trial (DCCT) results showed strict control of hyperglycemia in patients with type 1 diabetes without clinical neuropathy decreased the development of diabetic peripheral neuropathy 60% subjects (DCCT Trial, 1993). Animal research particularly on a rat model of type 1 diabetes (streptozotocin-induced) and spontaneous type 2 diabetes in Zucker fatty rats showed the best control of glycemic hypothesis with regard to neuropathy (Harwood Publishers, 2000 and Harwood Publishers, 2001). However, short life span of rodents severely limits the examination of chronic human diseases. Nonetheless, in general agreement with both clinical data of diabetic peripheral neuropathy and glycemic hypothesis, slowing sensory (Moore et al., 1980; Weis et al., 1995) and motor (Zochodne et al., 1994; Stevens et al., 2004) nerve conduction velocity that were shown to develop within the first month of onset of hyperglycaemia in diabetic rats.

2.5.2. Macrovascular Complications:

The underlying pathological mechanism in macrovascular disease is atherosclerosis which leads to narrowing of arteries throughout the body. Diabetes is also a strong independent predictor of risk of cerebrovascular and stroke as well as coronary artery disease. Diabetes increases the risk that an individual will develop cardiovascular disease (CVD) (Laing et al., 2003). CVD is the principal cause of death in people with either type 1 or type 2 diabetes (Laing et al., 2003; Paterson et al., 2007). CVD is the leading cause (~70%) of death in people with type 2 diabetes. A Worldwide Framingham study demonstrated the positive association of coronary heart disease with diabetes (Kannel et al., 1979). These findings have led to new guidelines and recommendations by American Diabetes Association and American Heart Association that diabetes is considered to be the major risk factor for coronary heart disease (Buse et al., 2005). Among people with type 2 diabetes, women may be at higher risk for coronary heart disease than men. The presence of microvascular disease is also a predictor of coronary heart events. People with diabetes (particularly T2DM) frequently have many traditional risk factors for CVD, including central obesity, dyslipidemia (i.e., elevated serum triglyceride, low-density lipoprotein (LDL), and free fatty acid levels and low high-density lipoprotein (HDL) levels), and hypertension (Leon et al., 2015). The combination of hyperglycemia, insulin resistance, dyslipidemia, hypertension, and chronic inflammation can injure the vascular endothelium, leading to macrovasculopathy and CVD in people with T2DM. Diabetes is an independent risk factor across all ages for stroke; the risk in people with diabetes is up to 2- to 4-fold greater. Patients with type 2 diabetes have a much higher risk of stroke, with an increased risk of 150–400%. The risk of stroke-related dementia and recurrence, as well as stroke-related mortality, is elevated in patients with diabetes. As in CVD, the presence of diabetes adversely affects the cerebrovascular circulation by increasing the risk of intracranial and extra-cranial (e.g., carotid artery) atherosclerosis (Beckman et al., 2012). People with diabetes have an increased incidence of traditional risk factors for stroke, including hypertension, dyslipidemia, heart failure, and atrial fibrillation. However, after these factors are controlled for, diabetes remains a strong predictor of stroke, suggesting that the presence of diabetes carries an independent risk for stroke apart from the increased presence of traditional risk factor. Insulin resistance is primarily associated with proatherogenic dyslipidemia as suggested by previous literature that showed hyperinsulinemia-induced activation of a hepatic SREBP-1 transcription factor involved in the prime event of insulin resistance mediaed via phosphatidylinositol 3-kinase (PI3K) (Shimomura et al., 1999 and Chen et al., 2007).

2.6. Diabetic Foot Ulcers:

DFU is a major secondary complication of diabetes, and impaired wound healing becomes limb and life threatening. The development of lower extremity ulcer among diabetics is the most important cause of morbidity and mortality. Once the ulcer develops, improper healing leads to wound progression causing amputation.

2.6.1. Epidemiology of Diabetic Foot Ulcers:

Both type 1 and type 2 diabetics are prone to develop foot ulcers, and about 85% of lower extremity amputations are preceded by non-healing foot ulcers (Rathur et al., 1990). The lifetime risk to a person with diabetes for developing a foot ulcer could be as high as 25% (Boyko et al., 1996). The rate of lower limb amputations is 15 times higher in diabetic patients compared with the non-diabetic patient. The annual population-based incidence of foot ulcer in people with type 1 or type 2 diabetes is from 1.9% to 2.2% (Ramsey et al., 1999). Foot problems in diabetic patients account for more hospital admissions than any other long-term complications of diabetes and also result in increasing morbidity and mortality. The diabetic foot syndrome encompasses a number of pathologies, including diabetic neuropathy, peripheral vascular disease, Charcot neuroarthropathy, foot ulceration, osteomyelitis, and the potentially preventable end point amputation. Patients with the diabetic foot can also have multiple diabetic complications and caring for such patients may require attention to many different areas. About 90,000 amputations per year as a result of non-traumatic diabetic foot complications (Joseph et al., 2003). A study reported that people of elder group are at a greater risk of developing foot ulcers and more susceptible to abscess and osteomyelitis (Reed et al., 2004). Developing regions face the biggest rise in the occurrence of type 2 diabetes in the next twenty years. Moreover, hence people of these countries will be disposed to ulceration (Boulton et al., 2005). The reported rate of foot ulcer prevalence was as high as 11.6 % by Centres for Disease Control and Prevention (CDCP) (2003) in United States. The 10.6% prevalence rate of DFU was reported in USA in a population-based study, with 2.2% an annual rate of incidence (Moss et al., 1992). In the same year, 7.4% prevalence rate of DFU was reported by Walter et al., 1992 in United Kingdom. Other reported rate of incidence was 1.8% in South Asia and 2.7% in African Caribbean and 5.5% in White Europeans (Abott et al., 2005). The average risk of foot ulcer development in peoples with diabetes is estimated to be 15% (Palumbo and Melton., 1995). The annual incidence of population -based studies has been summarized in Table 3.

Table 3: Selected population-based studies are estimating incidence and prevalence of DFUs.

Study (country)	Country	Population based	Annual Incidence	Prevalence	Ulcer definition	Method of ulcer assessment
Abott et al., 2005	United Kingdom	Registered T1 & T2 in 6 UK districts N=15,692	-	5.5% white european, 1.8% South Asian, 2.7% African Caribbean	Wagner grade ≥1 foot lesion	Clinical examination+chart review
CDCP	USA	US BRFSS	-	11.8(%)	Foot sore that did not heal for >4 weeks	Random digital telephonic
Kumal et al., 1994	UK	3 UK cities N=811	-	5.3(%)	NA	Direct xamination by expert
Moss et al., 1992	USA	Population-based study N=1834	2.2 (%)	10.6(%)	Full thickness skin loss on the foot	Medical history questionnaire and 4 years later
Muller et al., 2002	Netherland	Registered T2DM (1992-1998) N=3827	2.2 (%)	(7.4%)	Ulcer of lower leg	Abstracted medical record
Ramsey et al., 1999	USA	Registered T1DM & T2DM (1992-1995) N=8905	1.9 (%)		Wagner grade	Medical record
Walter et al., 1992	UK	Registered patient from 10 hospitals N=1077	-	7.4(%)	Wagner grade	Direct examination
Gadepalli et al., 2006	India	T1DM & T2DM, Hospital based(N=80)	-			Direct examination by expert

2.6.2. Pathogenesis of Diabetic Foot Ulcers:

DFU is an outcome of a complicated amalgam of various risk factors like peripheral neuropathy and ischemia from peripheral vascular disease (PVD) including other underlying causes involved such as deformed foot, trauma and impaired resistance to infection.

2.6.2.1. Diabetic Peripheral Neuropathy:

According to ADA (2005), diabetic neuropathy is defined as "the presence of symptoms and signs of peripheral nerve dysfunction in people with diabetes after exclusion of other causes. Neuropathy plays a pivotal role in diseases of the lower limb and associated disability. Diabetic peripheral neuropathy is considered as a frequent cause of disability of which early diagnosis is often overlooked. Upto 66% of patients with diabetes encounters peripheral neuropathy in the lower extremity. A population-based Rochester Diabetic Neuropathy Study conducted by epidemiologists of Mayo Clinic reported that between 60-65% of patients with either type 1 or type 2 diabetes had some kind of neuropathy (Zubair et al., 2010). However, no significant difference was obtained between the prevalence of neuropathy among the two diabetic groups. A longitudinal study from Finland reported the baseline prevalence of diabetic peripheral neuropathy to be 8.3% versus 2.1% in control group (Partanen et al., 1995). Some modifiable and non-modifiable risk factors account for development of diabetic peripheral neuropathy. Modifiable factors include hyperglycemia, hypertension, increased cholesterol levels and alcohol intake. Studies in animals as well as in vitro models reported that metabolic abnormalities caused due to hyperglycemia cause neuropathy (Tomlinson et al., 1998). In the development of neuropathy, the hyperglycemic state leads to an increase in the action of the enzymes aldose reductase and sorbitol dehydrogenase. This results in the conversion of intracellular glucose to sorbitol and fructose. The accumulation of these sugar products results in a decrease in the synthesis of nerve cell myoinositol, required for normal neuron conduction. Additionally, the chemical conversion of glucose results in a depletion of nicotinamide adenine dinucleotide phosphate stores, which are necessary for the detoxification of reactive oxygen species and he synthesis of the vasodilator nitric oxide (Yoshida et al., 1994). There is a resultant increase in oxidative stress in the nerve cell and an increase in vasoconstriction leading to ischemia, which will promote nerve cell injury and death. Hyperglycemia and oxidative stress also contribute to the abnormal glycation of nerve cell proteins and the inappropriate activation of PKC, resulting in further nerve dysfunction and ischemia. The diabetic control and complications trial and United Kingdom prospective diabetes study have demonstrated that good glycemic control prevents or slows down the progression of DPN. Non-modifiable factors encompass age, longer duration of diabetes, height and human leukocyte antigen - antigen D related (HLA-DR ¾) genotype (DCCT., 1998; UKPDS., 1993). These factors also play a major role in other microvascular complications of diabetes: nephropathy and retinopathy.

Neuropathy can be classified in various ways: Clinical presentation (symmetrical, focal, or painful, paralytic or ataxic), or on the basis of nerve fibers affected (motor, sensory, autonomic) or can be painful or without pain. In motor neuropathy damage to motor, nerves occur which effects body's ability to co-ordinate movements and leads to formation of foot deformity, Charcot's foot, hammerhead toes, and claws. Sensory neuropathy leads to damage of sensory nerves present in extremities. Ulcers caused by ill-fitting shoes, hurt by foreign objects, exposure to heat, etc are preceded by lack of sensations. Autonomic neuropathy leads to deportation in functions of sweat and sebaceous gland in foot causing a loss in natural moisturizing ability, the overlying skin and becomes dry and becomes more susceptible to tears and development of infection. Peripheral neuropathy in diabetes leads to structural alterations of foot leading to Charcot's foot, neuroarthropathy, osteoarthropathy and hammer head toes (Frykberg., 2010). Deep tissue infection reaching bone marrow (osteomyelitis) or cortex (osteitis) should be clinically examined by plain radiographs or magnetic resonance imaging.

*2.6.2.2. **Peripheral Vascular Disease (PVD):***

PVD is clinically defined as atherosclerotic occlusive diseases of lower limbs becoming a known marker for lower extremity loss, cerebro-vascular and cardiovascular diseases (Thiruvoipati et al., 2015). Peripheral dysfunction is diagnosed on the basis of diminished or absence of posterior or dorsal pedis pulses as well as medial arterial calcification. Progressive atherogenesis is a common event in patients with diabetes causing morbidity and mortality with health and wealth loss (Dhaliwal et al., 2007). All large vessels are involved followed by narrowing or thrombosis of cerebral, coronary, leg and renal vessels. PVD accounts for 70% death in T2DM. Approximately 20% of diabetics have an insufficient arterial blood supply. As reported in a recent study the peripheral arterial disease in diabetic subjects was more distal and poor outcome as compared to PVD in non-diabetics (Zubair et al., 2011). Ischemia of lower extremities as a consequence of proximal arterial disease is considered as major cause in pathways leading to diabetic foot ulcerations among 35% diabetic subjects in a 2 center study. The risk factors effecting PVD incidence include age, longer duration of diabetes, smoking habit, obesity and presence of peripheral neuropathy (Thiruvoipati et al., 2015). A cross-sectional study on 252 diabetic subjects reported altered lipid profile encompassing decreased HDL-cholesterol and elevated serum triglycerides. PVD is one of the important predisposing factors towards the development of foot ulcers in about 50% of cases (Beach et al., 1998). Approximately 20% of diabetics have an insufficient arterial blood supply. Many epidemiological studies have indicated hyperinsulinemia as independent risk factor for vascular diseases (Palumbo et al., 1995).

Atherosclerosis of arteries is a chronic inflammatory process later on getting converted into rupture of arteries. Fatty streaks formed by transportation and retention of lipoproteins in endothelial walls. Lipid oxidation in endothelium causes the release of chemoattractants which promotes the attraction of monocytes (Williams and Tabas., 1995). These inflammatory cells with enhanced oxidative capacity lead to further oxidation of lipoproteins entrapped in the endothelial wall. Highly oxidized lipoprotein particle is cytotoxic and taken up by recruited macrophages and conversion into foam cells, which is the hallmark of the atherosclerotic cascade. Diabetes enhances the transport of LDL in the endothelial wall and retention. In diabetes increased the permeability of endothelial wall that occurs in vessels exposed to hyperglycemia state. Increased advance glycation products (AGEs), a hallmark of diabetes covalently traps serum LDL leading to increased retention in sub-endothelium (Figure 8).

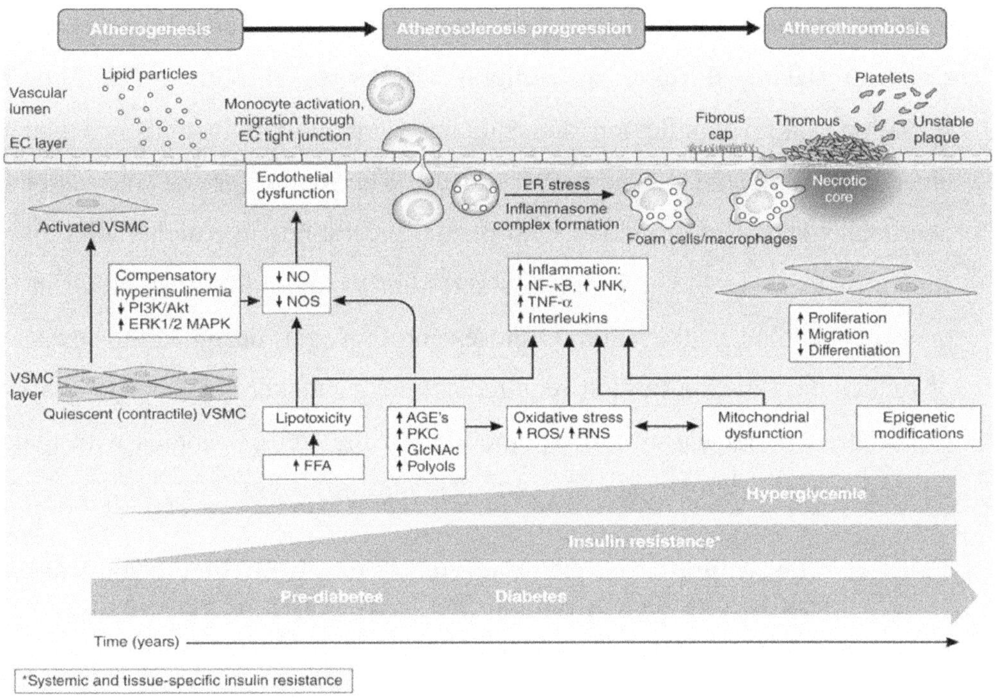

Figure 8: A postulate scheme for the mechanism of atherosclerosis in diabetes, emphasizing the role of glucose in the process.

*2.6.2.3. **Foot Biomechanics in Diabetes:***

Most of the injuries in diabetic foot with neuropathy occur in forefoot making an equal distribution in dorsal and plantar aspects. On the plantar and dorsal region sites of high pressure are prone to lesions making foot biomechanics as an essential contribute in ulcers (Edmonds et al., 1986). A pressure of 750 kPa will provide a cut-off value to differentiate between the low-risk and high-risk patient. The risk factors behind the biomechanics of diabetic foot include callus formation, thickened plantar tissues, and hindered joint mobility and foot deformities. Motor neuropathy causes imbalances in the flexor and extensor muscles of foot causing shifting of fat pad and prominent metatarsals heads and clawed toes causing an increase in load and pressure in diabetic foot. The etiology of callus is unrevealed, but as reported callus is responsible for sensation loss and frequent ulcerations. The etiology of callus is still unknown. In a study by Murray et al., 1996, the callus was present with the loss of sensation in foot, which have high risk of developing an ulcer. Therefore, it is strongly recommended to remove the callus from the foot using appropriate measures. Clinically it is therefore strongly suggested to remove callus formed. A significant co-relation between joint mobility at the subtalar joint and mobility at the first metatarsophalangeal joint. In addition, Muller et al., 2001, found decrease in sensation, ankle dorsiflexion and subtalar joint motion in diabetics patients with ulceration compared to normal controls. The demonstrated the association of neuropathy and joint limitation with plantar ulcerations in patients with diabetes. As shown by these studies, sensory loss and joint hypomobility may result in increased pressure and plantar ulceration. Orthoses and footwear, designed the stress over time or reduce the function motion requirements (e.g., rocker sole) during walking time, are needed to compensate for hypomobility in the feet of patients with hypomobilty (Hampton et al., 1990; Coleman., 1990; Thompson., 1988).

Table 4: "Two-minute foot examination" to check for biomechanical and other risk factors once a patient has been at risk of neuropathy or vascular disease.

Evaluation of component	Look for
Surface exam	Ulcer, callus. Hemorrhage in callus, blister, maceration between toe, breaks in skin, skin infection, edema, erythema, temperature
Nail exam	Fungal infection, ingrown toe nail, injury
Foot deformity	Prominent metatarsal head, clawed toes or hammertoes, rocker, bottom foot deformity, prior amputations
Examination of shoes	Drainage into socks, flatted insoles, leaning one side, poorly fitted.

2. 7. Classification of Diabetic Foot Ulcers:

Classification of foot wounds is needed to adequately describe the lesion to study patient's outcome. The system used should be clear, practical, relevant and easy to use. Each different class/ stage included should project a different diagnostic/ or therapeutic intervention so that it serves as a guide in clinical decision making. An adequate description of ulcer characteristics, such as size, depth, appearance, and location, also provides a mapping of progress during treatment. The evaluation should determine the etiology of the ulcer and ascertain whether the lesion is neuropathic, ischemic, or neuro-ischemic. Poor clinical results are associated with peripheral vascular disease, increasing wound depth and infection. It also appears that the progressive cumulative effect of these comorbidities contributes to a greater likelihood of a diabetic foot ulcer leading to a lower-limb amputation. Therefore a proper classification system is very important which can describe ulcer characteristics that will help in planning strategies for treatment of diabetic foot lesions.

Various classification systems have been implemented for determining the severity of diabetic foot lesions. The three most commonly used classification systems in diagnosis of diabetic foot lesions are discussed below:

1. Wagners- Meggitt Classification
2. University of Texas Classification
3. Depth Ischemia Classification
4. International Working Group Classification

2.7.1. Wagners- Meggitt Classification:

The most commonly used classification system developed in 1970 s by Wagner and Meggit. Though it was devised for dysvascular foot, it is in use since past 25 years. This classification system is universally accepted due to ease of use for investigators and clinicians. The system displays six grades, amongst them first four grades (0, I, II, III) are based on physical depth of wound in and through soft tissues of the foot, and last two grades (IV, V) are based on the extent of loss of perfusion in the foot. Wounds belonging to first four grades are pre-dominantly found, making deeper and advanced wounds of grade II and III prone to hospitalizations. Partial gangrene is a hallmark of grade IV and gangrene if entire foot describes grade V requiring amputation of gangrenous section of foot or limb. Though Wagner's grading is one of the most widely used classification system it does not take into consideration important clinical parameters such as ischemia, infection and other co-morbid factors (Wagner., 1981).

Table 5: Wagner-Meggitt Classification System (Wagners., 1981)

GRADE	FOOT LESION
0	No open lesions or cellulitis
I	Superficial ulcer
II	Deep ulcer upto tendons and joint tissue
III	Deep ulcer with abscess, osteomyelitis, and joint sepsis
IV	Local gangrene forefoot or heel
V	Gangrene of entire foot

2.7.2. Depth Ischemia Classification:

The depth ischemia classification system is a modified version of Wagner- Meggitt classification distinguishing between the evaluation of the wound and vascularity of foot, elucidate the distinctions among the grades and improvise the clinical co-relation of appropriate treatment of grades of lesions. The purpose of this system was to make classification more rational balance and easier. Diabetic foot wound is assigned number and letter grades and combination of both describe physical extent of wound (number) and ischemia or vascularity (number). The soft tissue section is inspected and graded with a number on the extent of depth, and next foot is evaluated for perfusion. The foot with grade 0 is considered to be at higher risk of post-ulcerations. A lesion of grade 1 is a superficial tear without exposure of deeper layers. Grade 3 lesions are deeper with exposed tendons or joint capsules with or without infection.

The deepest lesions belong to grade 3 with exposed infected bone, either abscess or osteomyelitis. The ischemia section of depth ischemia classification is defined by the letter A, B, C or D. Non- invasive vascular techniques such as Doppler Ultrasound or trans-cutaneous oxygen pressure are used to evaluate the foot for perfusion. The presence of bounding dorsal pedis or posterior tibial pulses is graded A without clinically significant ischemia. Grade C describes partial gangrene and grade D feet are completely gangrenous. The most common lesions belong to grade B which is ischemic but not gangrenous. The advantage of depth ischemia classification system is that it is succinct and once graded the treatment decisions becomes clear and concise (Brodsky et al., 1999).

Table 6: Depth Ischemic Classification System (Brodsky et al., 1999)

Depth		Ischaemia	
Grade	**Definition**	**Grade**	**Definition**
0	At risk, foot with previous ulcer that may cause new ulcer	**A**	No ischaemia
1	Superficial non-infected ulcer	**B**	Ischaemia no gangrene
2	Deep ulcer with tendon or joint exposed (+/- infection)	**C**	Partial forefoot gangrene
3	Extensive ulcer with bone exposed or deep abscess	**D**	Total foot gangrene

2.7.3. University of Texas Classification System (UTSA):

Wagner grading system is successfully modified by taking into considerations the parameters not included in Wagner's classification system. The University of Texas Antonio classification system assesses diabetic foot lesion according to depth, wound infection and the presence of lower limb ischemia. In this system grading is done on the basis of depth of the lesion and stages are classified on presence of ischemia, wound bioburden or combination of both excluding neuropathy (Oyibo et al., 2001). There are grades (0-3) and stages (A-D). Wounds of higher grade or stages are less prone to healing without vascular repair or lower extremity amputation. This system is superior in it outcomes as compared to Wagner grading. UTSA system is now widely used in various clinical trials and diabetic centers. Although the UTSA system (along with these others) recognizes the potential for infection at each of the different depths of ulcers, it goes no further in identifying the differences in organisms or needed antibiotic selection. Stage A has no ischemia or infection, stage B has an infection, stage has ischemia and stage D has both ischemia and infection (Armstrong et al., 1998).

Table 7: University of Texas Classification System (Armstromg et al., 1998)

Stages	Grades 0	1	2	3
A	Healed pre or post ulcerative lesion completely epithelialized	Superficial wound not involving bone tendon or capsule	Wound penetrating tendon and capsule	Wound penetrating to bone or joint
B	With infection	With infection	With infection	With infection
C	With ischemia	With ischemia	With ischemia	With ischemia
D	With infection and With ischemia	With infection and With ischemia	With infection and With ischemia	With infection and With ischemia

2.7.4. International Working Group Classification (IWDGF):

Another classification system given by International Working Group that gives information about risk that can predict which people with diabetes are at risk for diabetes foot problems. The risk assessment instrument developed by the International Working Group on the Diabetic Foot (IWGDF) has been shown to predict diabetic foot complications (Peters et al., 2001).

Table 8: International Working group on the Diabetic Foot (Peters et al., 2001)

Group	Definition
Risk group 0	No neuropathy, no PVD
Risk Group 1	No neuropathy, no PVD
Risk Group 2	Neuropathy and deformity and or PVD
Risk Group 3	History Pathology

2.8. Lower Limb Amputation in Diabetic Foot Patients:

The amputation rate varies across the geographical locations within the country and or within the countries. The *Global Lower Extremity Amputation Study Group* first time reported the rate of amputation in lower limb in diabetic subjects, pooling a data from the 10 study centres over a period of 2 years in USA. They reported a lowest rate 2.8 per 100,000 persons per year in Madrid, Spain and the highest in Navojo population with a rate of amputation as 43.9 per 100,000 per year (Gleasg., 2000). The annual incidence of amputation has been shown in table 06. The annual incidences of amputation were changes from 0.7 per 1000 in East Asia to 31.0 per 1000 in USA (Moss et al., 1999, Humphrey et al., 1966, Humphrey et al., 1994, Lehto et al., 1996, Trautner et al., 1996). Lower Extremity Amputation (LEA) rates can be 15 to 40 times higher among the diabetic versus non diabetic populations (ADA., 1999; Larvey et. al., 1996; Frykberg., 1999; Resnick et al., 1999, Viswanathan and Kumpatla., 2011). It was estimated that every 30 second, amputation was done due to diabetes somewhere in the world (Viswanathan and Kumpatla., 2011). It was also suggested that, amputation was done for disease management and remained a global problem for all persons with diabetes (Jefficoate., 2005). The same risk factors that predispose to ulceration can also generally be considered contributing causes of amputation, albeit with several modifications. Another frequently described risk factor for amputation is chronic hyperglycemia. Results of the Diabetes Control and Complications Trial DCCT and the United Kingdom Prospective Diabetes Study (UKPDS) support the long held theory that chronic poor control of diabetes is associated with a host of systemic complications (DCCT., 1993; UKPDS., 1998). The best predictor for amputation is a history of previous amputation. A past history of a lower extremity ulceration or amputation increases the risk for further ulceration, infection, and subsequent amputation (Harris., 1998; Larsson et. al., 1998; Boyko et. al., 1999; Adler et. al., 1999). It may also be inferred that patients with previous ulceration possess all the risk factors for developing ulceration, having demonstrated that they already have the component elements in the causal pathway (Reiber et. al., 1995; Frykberg, 1998; Larvey et. al., 1998). Up to 34% of patients develop another ulcer within 1 year after healing an index wound, and 5 year rate of developing a new ulcer is 70% (Apleqvist et al., 1993; Larsson et. al., 1995). Re- amputation can be attributed to disease progression, non-healing wounds, and additional risk factors for limb loss that develop as a result of the first amputation. Tragically, the 5 year survival rate after a diabetes related LEA has been reported to be as low as 28% to 31% (Ebskov., 1998). One study reported a 5 year mortality rate of 68% after lower limb amputation, with lower survival rates in those patients with higher levels of amputation. Persons with renal failure or more proximal levels of amputation have a poor prognosis and higher mortality rate. Those who undergo a diabetes- related amputation have a 40% to 50% chance of undergoing a contralateral amputation within 2 years (Tentolouris., 2004). Population based study of diabetic individuals with non-traumatic amputations from the US hospitals were the three main well known geographical risk factors: age, gender and non-white racial status. In the year 2003, there was an increase in amputation rate by 2 fold in those who were at the age of ≥75 years (CDCP). The importance of quality of easily assessable care clinic and socio-economic of patients were also important significant factors in deciding the rate of amputations (Nielsen et al., 1998; Resnick et al., 1999; Abbas et al., 2005). The peripheral neuropathy is also associated with the amputation risk. These includes insensitivity to 10g monofilament, decrease motor nerve conduction velocity of the deep peroneal nerve and sensory nerve conduction velocity ofthe sural nerve, VPT, absent or diminished bilateral vibration sensation, and absent Achilles tendon and patellar reflexes. Table 07 shows the studies that reported a statistically significant association between one or more measures of peripheral neuropathy and amputation (Lehto et al., 1996; Nelson et al., 1988; Reiber et al., 1992, Selby and Zhang, 1995; Adler et al., 1999, Hamalainen et al., 1999; Selby et al., 2001; Mayfield et al., 1996; Adler et al., 1999; Hamalainen et al., 1999; Mayfield et al., 1996; Hennis et al., 2004; Selby et al., 2001). The studies done by Moss et al., 1999 and Resnick et al., 2004 did not show any association with the amputation and peripheral neuropathy. The peripheral arterial function, as measured by absent or diminished dorsal pedis and posterior tibialis pulses as well as median arterial calcification and its relationship to amputations, is an independent risk factors to predict the amputation in diabetic patients with foot ulcer (Lehto et al., 1996; Nelson et al., 1988; Reiber et al., 1992; Adler et al., 1999; Hamalainen et al., 1999; Mayfield et al., 1996; Hennis et al., 2004; Resnick et al., 2004). High blood pressure is also an independent predictive risk factor for amputation in various studies (Moss et al., 1999; Selby & Zhang., 1995; Lee et al., 1993). Six studies have reported no significant role of high blood pressure with amputation rate in their final outcome (Lehto et al., 1996, Nelson et al., 1988; Reiber et al., 1992; Hamalainen et al., 1999; Mayfield et al., 1996; Hennis et al., 2004). High BP was the significant factor in males and elevated diastolic BP in females for amputation (Lee et al., 1993). Long duration of diabetes is also significantly associated with amputation (Moss et al., 1999; Lehto et al., 1996; Nelson et al., 1988; Selby and Zhang., 1995; Adler et al., 1999; Hamalainen et al., 1999; Selby et al., 2001, Mayfield et al., 1996; Lee et al., 1993; Hennis et al., 2004; Resnick et al., 2004). Poor glycemic control as measured by elevated HbA1c with or without plasma glucose reported to be an important risk factors for increased risk of amputation in a nine analytical studies represented in table 7. Smoking was an independent risk factor for increased risk of amputation in diabetic patients (Moss et al., 1999) and also the patients with history of prior foot ulcer, an independent risk factor (Moss et al., 1999; Adler et al., 1999; Mayfield et al., 1996). There is a statistical significant association between the risk of amputation and presence of retinopathy (Moss et al., 1999; Lehto et al., 1996; Nelson et al., 1988; Reiber et al., 1992; Selby and Zhang, 1995; Hamalainen et al., 1999; Mayfield et al., 1996; Lee et al., 1993).

2.9. Wound Healing In Diabetic Foot Ulcers:

The healing of diabetic wound is a complex mechanism which involves an intricately regulated sequence of cellular and biochemical events orchestrated to restore tissue integrity after injury (Figure 9). Each of these phases is controlled by biologically active agents called growth factors. Growth factors are hormone-like polypeptides, present in very small amounts in the body that control the growth, differentiation, and metabolism of cells. The wound healing process involves the three distinct but overlapping phases (Figure 9).

(i) Hemostasis and inflammation **(ii) Proliferation**

(iii) Maturation and Remodeling

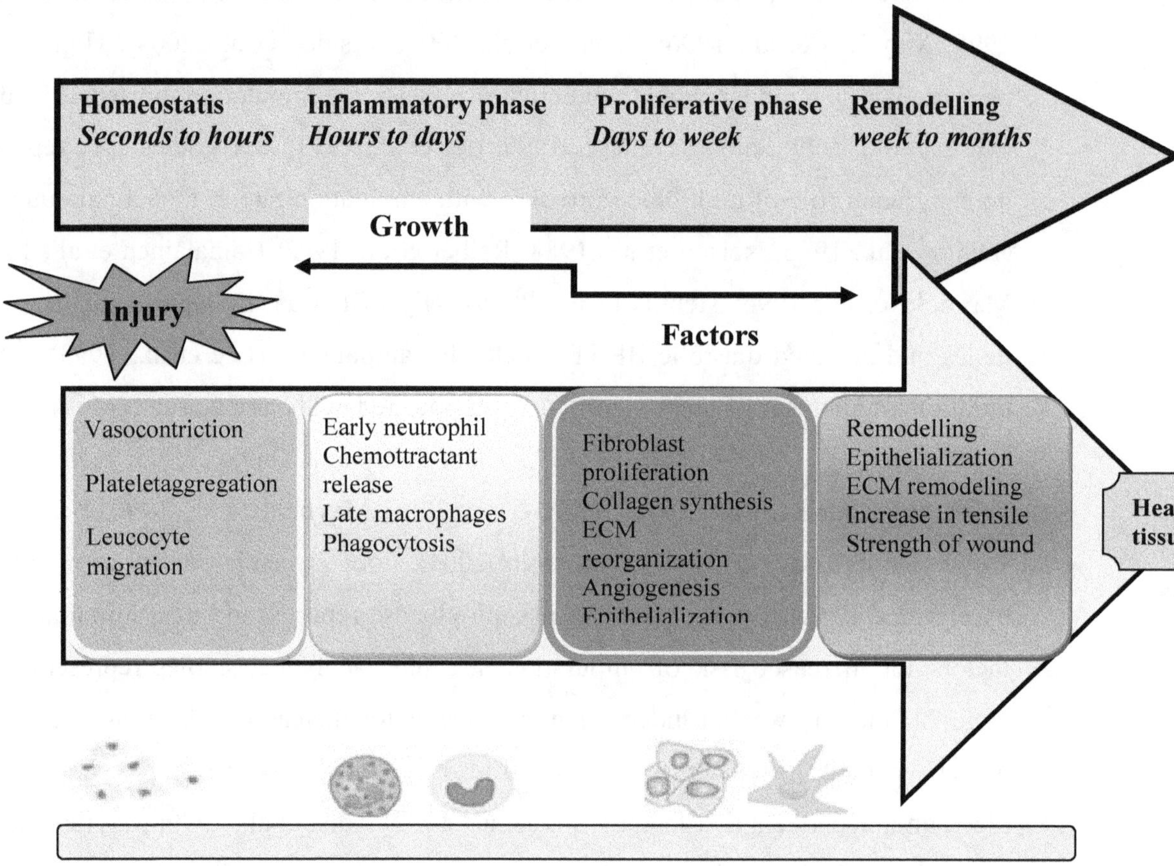

Figure 9: Distinct and overlapping phases of wound healing (Current concepts of in the physiology of adult wound healing (Meethale et al., 2015).

2.9.1. Homeostasis and Inflammation:

Homeostasis follows the traumatic rupture of blood vessels exposed to subendothelial collagen and platelets leading to the activation of intrinsic part of the coagulation cascade (Witti and Barbul., 1997). The inflammation is characterized by increased in vascular permeability, poly-morphonuclear cells (chemotaxis) from circulation into the wound and it activates the migrating cells. The neutrophils are the first to arrive at the site of wound and its role is primary phagocytic and wound debridement and it is a source of proinflammatory cytokines which serve to activation of the local fibroblast and keratinocytes (Park and Barbul., 2004; Hubner et al., 1996). It decreases the infection in wound (Simpson and Ross., 1972), as they are not essential because their role in phagocytosis and antimicrobial defense are taken up by macrophages. The macrophage will migrate to into wound 48-98 hrs after injury and participate in the inflammatory process. Their antimicrobial functions will include phagocytosis and generation of reactive free radicals, such as nitric oxide, oxygen, and peroxide. It develops functional complement receptors and undertakes similar operations to the neutrophil (Cherry et al., 2000). The wound healing is severely impaired if macrophage infiltration of the wound is prevented.

2.9.2. Proliferation:

The new tissue matrix are essential for physical support for new blood vessel, arising from the intact vasculature in the surrounding dermis, and angiogenesis is critical to provide the basic nutrient and oxygen which help in synthesis of collagen. Hence collagen and capillary proliferation occur in a co-dependent manner. During this phase, fibroblast, and endothelial cells are primary cells that multiply in this process. Fibroblast responsible for replacing the fibrin matrix called clot and also produce and release proteoglycans and glycosaminoglycans, an extra-component for tissue granulation. The fibroblast production will stop when sufficient collagen was produced. During healing and repair, angiogenesis a fundamental biological mechanism is activated (Carmeliet., 2005), which is characterized by invasion, migration, and proliferation of endothelial cells and those which are close to side walls of vessel start migration because of angiogenesis. The cytoplasmic pseudopods start sprouting in wound and forms perivascular space, and the endothelial cells also proliferate to cell migration and produce degradation enzyme. Several biological factors like, platelets, macrophages, lymphocyte, keratinocyte production (fibroblast growth factor α and β, transforming growth factor α & β, epidermal growth factor, hepatocyte growth factor and IL-1) are reported to be potent stimuli for new vessel formation (Grant et al., 1993). Hypoxia (create oxygen granulation), lactate and extracellular matrix also mediate cell growth. Several adhesive proteins like

Willebrand factor, fibrinogen, fibronectin up-regulate the α & β integrin adhesive receptors. These integrin factors initiate the calcium-dependent signaling pathways leading to cell migration. Once the wound is filled with new granulation tissue, angiogenesis stops, and many vessels disintegrate as a result of apoptosis.

2.9.3. Maturation and Remodeling:

The main feature in the maturation phase is collagen deposition in wound space. The rate of maturation, quality and the total amount of matrix deposition determine the strength of scar. To support the future matrix deposition and remodelling, glycosaminoglycans and proteoglycans are synthesized (Witte and Barbul., 1997). The collagen is a predominant scar protein, and extracellular matrix components are remodeled by matrix metalloproteinases. The source of collagenases in the wound is the inflammatory cells and endothelial cells as well as fibroblast and keratinocyte. These can degenerate, and the activity of collagen was tightly controlled by cytokines.

2.10. Infection in Diabetic Foot Ulcers:

Many types of infection, mostly bacterial are common in diabetic patients (Viswanathan et al., 2011). Soft tissue and foot infections are considered as the most frequent types in diabetics. Foot infections are the most common of all with devastating outcomes. Development of infection after ulceration is a pivotal event for gradual tissue necrosis. The severity of DFIs ranges from mild to limb or life threatening. Infection is not the cause rather a consequence of DFUs. All infections begin as a slight problem may progress to involve deep tissues, joints, or bones especially if not managed. The infection complicates the pathological picture of diabetic foot. Infection also plays a critical role in formation of moist gangrene. DFI and their outcomes are associated with acute or long-term morbidity including the need of surgical treatments or amputations.

2.10.1. Epidemiology of Diabetic Foot Infection:

A large retrospective study done in Canada reported that nearly half of population suffering from diabetes gets hospitalized for infectious disease in a year (Shah et al., 2003). The frequency of foot cellulitis was found to be nine times greater in diabetic subjects when compared with non-diabetics) whereas foot osteomyelitis is responsible for 12 times greater hospitalizations in diabetic subjects than in non-diabetic people in diabetics (Boyko and Lipsky., 2004)). Study on DFUs reported that the presence of infection increases the risk of a lower extremity amputation by 50% compared to ulcer patients without infection. A two-year longitudinal study done in Texas reveals that among 1666 diabetic patients enrolled 151 (9.1%) patients developed 199 infected foot ulcers (Lavery et al., 2006). Most of the clinical and retrospective studies explored that 25% to 50% of DFIs causes minor surgical amputations and 10% to 40% requires major amputations (IWGDF, 1999). Therefore, infection preceded by ulcers is often proximate causes of deadly outcomes. Around 60% of infected foot ulcers are headed by loss of lower limb, and becomes one of awful outcomes in diabetic foot patients (Pecoraro et al., 1991; Reiber et al., 1992). The independent risk factors were found to be, wounds involving bone, ulcer duration of > 30 days, recurrent ulcers, and the presence of PVD.

2.10.2. Risk factors:

A blend of physiologic and metabolic factors places diabetic patients at a high risk for foot wounds invaded by infections. Various predisposing factors, including neuropathy, delayed wound healing, and vasculopathy lies behind infected ulcers. Immunological defects associated with diabetes in the host such as impaired polymorphonuclear leukocytes functions, abnormalities in phagocytosis and intracellular killings are directly related to metabolic perturbations caused by poorly controlled hyperglycemia.

Persistent abscesses and poor granulation of tissues accompanied by impaired wound healing predispose to infected foot ulcers. *Staphylococcus aureus* is predominant on the skin of diabetic patients and invades when dermal surface breaks down. Skin harbored by fungal infection breaks cutaneous envelope, forming potential sites for bacterial invasion.

Anatomical modification in the structure of diabetic foot, including tendons, neurovascular bundles favors the spread of infection. Edema with acute infection elevates compartment pressure associated with rigid and bony structures of medial, central and lateral sections of foot, causing ischemic necrosis of tissues.

2.10.3. Diagnosis of Infection in Diabetic Foot Ulcers:

Infection is diagnosed clinically not microbiologically. Ulceration or sores in skin are beginning regions for infection in diabetics. Though most of the infections remain superficial such as simple cellulitis, and around 25% will spread from epidermal layer to deeper regions involving subcutaneous tissues and bones such as septic arthritis, necrotic fasculitis and Osteomyelitis (Lipsky et al., 2004). Wound infections must be diagnosed clinically on the basis of local and occasionally systemic signs and symptoms of inflammation. According to the Infectious Disease Society of America (IDSA) guidelines, infection is present if there is obvious purulent drainage and the presence of two or more signs of inflammation (erythema, pain, tenderness, warmth, or induration. Diagnosis of foot ulcers in diabetics is done by the presence pus secretion from an infected wound and certain physical factors including erythema, tenderness, and pain.

2.10.4. Assessment of Severity of Infection:

Clinical assessment requires appropriate debridement to remove necrotic sections and callus to fully visualize the wound. Infection should be initially accessed first by appearance of a local foot problem or signs of inflammation (swelling, redness, sinus tract or crepitation) a systemic infection (eg rigor, vomiting, tachycardia, confusion malaise and fever) or a metabolic disorder (severe hyperglycemia, ketosis and azotemia). It should be considered when the local signs are less severe than expected (Williams et al., 2004). Assessment of severity of infection is essential in selecting the appropriate antibiotic which influences the route of drug administration and need for hospitalization and potential necessity and timing of surgical proceedings. Evaluation of infection severity is essential in selection of antibiotic regime. This also helps in assessing the potential need of surgical treatment.

Table 9: Clinical characteristics that help to define the severity of infection

Features	Mild Infection	Serious Infection
Presentation	Slowly progressive	Acute or rapidly progressive
Ulceration	Involves skin only	Penetration to subcutaneous tissue
Tissue involved	Epidermal and dermal	Fascia, muscle, tendon, joint, bone
Cellulitis	Minimal (<2 cm ring)	Extensive, or distant from ulceration
Local signs	Slight inflammation	Severe inflammation, crepitus, bullae
Systemic signs	None or minimal	Fever, chills, hypotension, confusion, volume depletion, leukocytosis
Metabolic control	Mildly abnormal	Severe hyperglycemia, acidosis, azotemia
Foot vasculature	Minimal impaired	Absent pulse, reduced ankle and toe blood pressure
Complicating features	None or minimal	Gangrene, Escher, foreign body, abscess, marked edema, osteomyelitis

2.10.5. Microbiology of Diabetic Foot Infection:

Infection is said to occur when virulent organisms invade the body, overpowers host defense and leads to local tissue damage. The skin is coated with normal flora present in harmless association either present permanently or transient. *Staphylococcus aureus* and *beta-hemolytic cocci* are rarely found on intact skin but may be present transiently, rapidly colonizing disrupted epithelium. The destruction of local tissues followed by multiplication of microbes the lesion is infected. Infection encompasses invasion of microbes in host tissues by pathogens, followed by host immune response. Superficial infection is restricted to soft tissue (skin or subcutaneous surface) while deeper infections involve tendons, joints or bones. Infection in diabetic foot can be caused by a single microorganism (mono-microbial) or more than one (poly-microbial). Ulcers infected for shorter duration are mono-microbial and invaded by gram-positive pathogens (Lipsky et al., 1990). Chronic and long-standing wounds are polymicrobial and develop complex flora with gram-negative aerobes, anaerobes and *Enterococci*.

The normal skin flora includes gram-positive aerobes, *α- hemolytic streptococci*, or *corneybacteria*. However, the colonizing flora becomes more complex notably *Staphylococcus aureus* and *β hemolytic cocci*, in diseases like psoriasis and diabetes.

2.10.6. Etiology of Microbial Profile:

Various aspects of wound microbiology are responsible for development of foot infection. These include microbial load, microbial diversity, and presence of infective organisms and synergistic relationship between microbial species. Infection is said to occur when microbial load is greater than 10^5 organisms per gram of tissue.

Several microorganisms have been evaluated in microbial etiology of infected foot ulcers. These ranges from aerobic to anaerobic species and fungi. Potential (latent) pathogens of the DFU are believed to include *Staphylococcus*, *Streptococcus*, *Proteobacteria*, *Pseudomonas aureginosa* and *coliform* bacteria (Smith et al., 2016). *Staphylococcus aureus* and *beta-hemolytic cocci* are also the most frequently isolated microbes in DFI. *Staphylococcus aureus* has been reported in frequencies varying from 43% of infected foot ulcer (Hansson et al., 1995). *Pseudomonas aeuroginosa* is another frequently identified organism and has been found in 7–33% of ulcer (Urbancic et al., 1997). Foot ulcers with ischemia and deep tissue necrosis are reported to have anaerobic growth (Zubair et al., 2010). Chronic infected foot ulcers often show poly-microbial growth, including gram-negative rods or anaerobes, obligate anaerobes and *enterococci* (Frykberg., 2003). Severe cases of diabetic foot contain poly-microbial isolates. Whereas, in most of the mild infections mono-microbial pattern is found (Frykber., 2003). Cultures of specimens obtained from patients with mixed infections yield 3–5 isolates, including gram-positive and gram-negative aerobes and anaerobes (Armstrong et al., 1995; Golstein et al., 1996).

Furthermore some studies suggest that the interactions of organisms within these poly-microbial mixtures lead to the production of virulence factors, such as collagenases, proteases, and hemolysins, as well as short-chain fatty acids, that cause inflammation, obstructed wound healing, and contribute to the chronicity of the infection (Citron et al., 2007). Many studies from western countries reported that predominant organism isolated from DFI is gram positive aerobes (Dang et al., 2003). Whereas several studies from Eastern countries have reported the presence of gram-negative aerobes as predominant organisms. In a study, the prevalence of pathogens in DFI about parameters such as Wagner's grading, duration of diabetes, and healing times was studied. It was found that in 654 diabetic patients, 728 pathogens were isolated. Aerobic pathogens were isolated in 66.8% patients, and anaerobic pathogens were isolated in 33.2%. As Wagner's grading increased, the prevalence of anaerobic pathogens also increased (Viswanathan et al., 2002).

The first poly-microbial study on DFI done in Boston USA in 1976 reported the presence of major pathogens *Bacteroides species* (14.6%), followed by *Peptococci species* (13.7%), *Proteus species* (9.4%), *Enterococcus* species (7.7%), *Staphylococcus aureus* (7.7%), *Clostridium species* (7.7%) and *Escherichia coli* (7.0%) (Louie et al., 1976). On an average, about 5.2 organisms per patient were reported. A quantitative study conducted by Sapico et al., 1980, on 13 DFU patients in California, USA reported the presence of aerobic (51.7%) and anaerobic (43.1%), and only 5.1% were fungal pathogens. In this study, 4.7 strains per patients were found. In the year 1996, another study by Tan et al., 1996, in Ohio, a total of 112 DFU patients were studied. *Staphylococcus species* were the most common single organisms isolated. *Corynebacterium* isolates were usually found as one of multiple organisms. 92% of the pathogens were aerobic organisms among them 67% were gram-positive cocci in a study done by Lipsky et al. in 1997. The most commonly isolated organism among all patients was *Proteus mirabilis* (13%), *Enterococcus species* and *Escherichia coli* (12% each respectively) Among the anaerobic microbes, 26.7% were *Peptostreptococcus species*, followed by *Actinomyces Israelis* (13.3%), *Bifidobacterium species* and *Clostridium species* (10.0% each). Anandi et al., (2004) studied the bacterial etiology of 107 DFU patients from India. The most common aerobic bacteria was *Escherichia coli* (27.7%) followed by *Proteus species* (16.9%), *Staphylococcus aureus* and *Klebsiella species* (13.6% each). The commonest among anaerobes was *Clostridium species* (60%), followed by *Bacteroides fragilis* (20%), *Prevotella species* (13.3%) and *Peptostreptococcus species* (6.7%).

A study by Abdulrazak et al., 2005, on 86 DFU patients from Kuwait showed the presence of both anaerobic and anaerobic isolates. The most commonly isolated aerobic bacterial species were *Staphylococcus aureus* (38.4%), *Pseudomonas aeruginosa* (17.5%), and *Proteus mirabilis* (14%). Among anaerobic infection, the most frequently isolated bacteria were *Bacteroides fragile* and the fungal infection was represented by 7%. In France, Sotto et al., 2007, studied 173 DFU patients and found that polymicrobial infection was found in 73.9% cases and 24.8% cases were monomicrobial. Among Gram-positive cocci staphylococcus was most commonly found (38.1%) and among aerobic gram-negative *Enterobacteriaceae* were the most frequent pathogens.

In Malaysia, Raja., 2007, from Malaysia, recovered 287 microbes from 194 DFU patients The organisms isolated were *Staphylococcus aureus* (17%) followed by *Proteus* species (15%), *Pseudomonas aeruginosa* (13%), *Group B Streptococcus* (11%) and *Bacteroides species* (1%). Amongst anaerobes were isolated, *Peptotreptococcus species*, *Bacteroides species* and *Clostridium species, Candida species* (0.69%) were also isolated. Lily et al., 1999, conducted a study and reported the presence of anaerobic organisms. The isolates were *Peptostreptococcus species* (47%) and Bacteroides fragilis group (19%), *Prevotella species* (3%), *Clostridium species* (2%), *Fusobacterium species* (2%), *Eggerthella species* and *Acidominococcus species* (1% each respectively). Ramakant et al., 2011, studied the changing microbiological profile of pathogenic bacteria isolated from DFU in Northern India period of 8 years. In their study, they reported that Gram-negative bacterial infection was increasing from 50.6% to 66%. The most common isolate was Pseudomonas aeruginosa (16.9%) followed by *Eschirechia coli* (16.1%) and Proteus spp. (8.8%).

Other Gram-negative aerobes recovered were *Citrobacter species*, *Enterobacter species* and *Acinetobacter*.

2.10.7. Antibiotic Resistance in Diabetic Foot Pathogens:

The infection of DFU and the résistance to drugs of various classes in this group of patients is a central and major health issue which needs to be addressed. The problem of increasing diabetic population and subsequently ulcer, along with the increasing prevalence of antibiotic resistance, makes this highly pertinent issue a major area of concern. Moreover, the polymicrobial nature is likely to provide an appropriate environment for genetic exchange between bacteria making these problems worse. Different populations suffering from DFU show wide variation in the intensity of antibiotic resistance. A prospective study of uninfected chronic venous leg ulcer from 66 patients who had received no antibiotics in the previous month showed a very low level of antibiotic resistance, only two patients were found to have MRSA (Davies et al., 2003). Day and Armstrong, 1997, reviewed the limited evidence on risk factors for the carriage of resistance in diabetic foot wounds. While they found no studies that had directly addressed this issue, suggested risks include cross-contamination of wounds from the patients themselves, inanimate objects or health care personnel, long-term use of antibiotics, prior hospitalization and severity of illness. High prevalence of antibiotic resistance, especially MRSA, affects treatment decisions concerning wounds and raises the question of whether the empirical regimens could cover these resistant organisms (Armstrong et al., 2004). Whilst the additional impact of antibiotic-resistant organisms on wound healing is not known, overall, the morbidity, mortality and cost associated with infections in hospitalised patients caused by antibiotic-resistant organisms has been shown to be 1.3- to 2-fold higher than those infections caused by antibiotic-sensitive organisms (Howell Jones et al., 2005).

2.10.8. Laboratory Diagnosis of Infection:

Culturing of clinically uninfected wound is unnecessary unless it is required for the epidemiological purpose. Defining the microbiological cause in infected foot will usually assist in subsequent management of infection. A culture of samples will identify the microbes present in infection, but only if the specimens are collected properly and processed according to recommended guidelines. Usually the patients with severe long standing diabetes, complicated foot and previous antibiotic use will have polymicrobial infection in their wound. Culture specimens are sometimes defined by how results are reliable (Wheat et al., 1986). The patients with diabetic foot ulcerations with infection enforce a severe burden despite of all preventive measures. Hence, isolation and identification of causative microorganism is necessary in DFIs. There are four techniques commonly used for sample collection from wound of diabetic foot patients including aspiration, swab, tissue biopsy and curettage. Tissue biopsy is known as the most advantageous and standard method according to several studies, but due to increased possibility of spreading infection, loss of adjacent structure in limb and ischemia tissue biopsy is not advisable. Swab cultures are manageable since collection becomes easier from any kind of wound. However, swab cultures are sometimes not dependable since they generally include the colonizers and not the causative pathogen. Even now results of swab cultures are being extensively used methods for identification of causative pathogen and selection of antibiotic. Culturing technique therefore plays an important role bacterial identification.

2.10.8.1. Conventional Microbiology

Chronic wounds or wounds that fail to progress through normal wound healing trajectory or wounds with severe infections are imposing great burden on an already burdened healthcare system. These long-standing lesions found in (DFUs, venous leg ulcers, pressure sores, non-healing surgical wounds) are all increasing at alarming rates due to inactive lifestyles, obesity, lack of physical exercise and, most importantly, unbound increase in diabetes every year. The untreatable infected wound leads to loss of lower extremity, patient eventually loss of life for far too many patients. A possible reason for such severe condition is unmanageable treatment methodologies, wrong antimicrobial therapy, and delayed wound healing, improper evaluation of wound bio-burden. Conventional techniques rely on traditional bacteriological methodologies for evaluation of wound microbial flora. Traditional clinical culture techniques are widely used diagnostic tools available.

The specimens for culture are obtained after washing the wound vigorously with saline followed by debridement of superficial exudates. In bacteriological assays specimens are promptly sent to microbiology lab for identification of causative pathogens (Gadepalli et al., 2006). It is rational to consider that improving the methods of microbial detection and identification may prove successful in helping the clinician deal with this important healthcare problem. Furthermore, an organism which colonizes the tissue becomes difficult to isolate. Using conventional techniques, the mean number of bacterial species per ulcer has been found to range from 1.6 up to 4.4. Hansson et al., 1995, observed that 86% of ulcers with no clinical signs of infection contained more than one bacterial species. Previous studies have compared culturing to molecular methods. Moreover, these studies have reported that molecular techniques are more sensitive and reliable then culture methods and hold a promise for patient care (Dowd et al., 2008). A wide range of microbial diversity can be exposed in a single wound sample by using culture free sequencing of bacterial DNA (Findley et al., 2013).

2.10.9. Molecular Approaches:

The deoxy-ribonucleic acid (DNA) structure was given in late 1960 s, and routinely brought in use after the discovery of restriction enzymes and various genomic techniques. Recent advances in molecular/genome associated methods have revolutionized the evaluation and characterization of microorganisms in a broad range of medical diagnostic areas, including, mycology, parasitology, virology, dentistry and microbiology (Valones et al., 2009). Over past 20 years, the use of nucleic acid amplification technology in field of microbiology has exposed unanswered questions. Nowadays, molecular detection techniques especially polymerase chain reaction (PCR) based, have become an innovative and specific method for pathogen identification in clinical diagnostic laboratory setting (Bowler et al., 1999; Dowd et al., 2008).

Exploring the microbial profile using traditional conventional methodologies takes in several days for sufficient growth for accurate detection. In clinical diagnosis, a delay in obtaining results may pose a serious burden on patient management causing empirical treatment.

PCR-based methods should be incorporated to identify the causative pathogen which is fastidious or slow growing and cannot be identified by conventional methods (Speers., 2006). Development of drug resistance in isolated pathogens has become an important issue making the treatment extremely difficult. PCR-based assays can be implied in the detection of multi-drug resistant genes in a shorter span of time. MRSA can be identified by simple PCR assay by targeting *mec*A gene. The array of pathogens in wounds of patients can be more easily and sensitively explored by using molecular methodologies than culture-based technique (Melendez et al., 2010). Molecular tools cannot be used in quantitative estimation such as microbial load or number. Determination of true causative agent in necessary, therefore, use of molecular techniques enables a full identification of the microbiota within an infected diabetic ulcer (Lavigne et al., 2015).

2.10.9.1. <u>Use of PCR in Bacterial Identification</u>

PCR was developed in the 1980s by Kary Mullis, and awarded the Nobel Prize in 1994, This technology has caused a absolute revolution in biological research, establishing the agreement of basic biological processes in applied regions involving diagnoses and genetic improvements for plants and animal. PCR amplifies specific DNA regions using a DNA-polymerase enzyme, which takes part in the replication of the cellular genetic material. PCR is in-vitro presentation of natural genetic replication occurring in the cells, synthesizing complementary genetic sequences. A set of primer, a small section of DNA complementary to specific site to start synthesis is connected to one of the strands.

To exhibit the role of pathogens in wound infection, it is important to define the full array of organisms within a wound. A highly organized arrangement of bacterial communities is called as biofilm (Davey et al., 2000). Formation of biofilms is another factor which leads to chronicity of diabetic foot wound. Biofilms are cooperative communities of sessile bacteria that are rooted in an extra polysaccharide matrix with transformed phenotype and growth patterns (Dang et al., 2016). It therefore, becomes necessary to uncover the physiological arrangements of bacteria in biofilms of diabetic foot wounds which due to lack of technologies remains unexplored. Genomic tools such as amplification of nucleic acids, DNA sequencing such as denaturing gradient gel elecrophoresis (DGGE) and pyrosequencing, and development of 16S ribosomal clone libraries have transfigured the potential to understand the microbiology of wounds (Martin et al., 2010), and may also recast approaches to the use of antimicrobial agents in the treatment of infected diabetic wounds. In addition to it the large numbers of micro-organisms that are fastidious or non-cultivable in traditional conventional methods are also revealed (Pongsachareonnont et al., 2017). This fundamental information obtained by the results of molecular techniques can be linked to clinical course for treatment methodologies. Furthermore, species-specific sequences, which are analyzed to detect individual bacterial species, are typically found adjacent to the 16S ribosomal DNA. For the identification of bacterial DNA in the specimen, amplification of 16S DNA is done, which identifies the bacterial DNA, and then the flanking sequences are identified and compared with a known library of bacterial sequences, which then identifies the species (Knox et al., 1998). Genomic techniques have the aptitude to overcome the bacterial sampling problems that are often encountered in infected diabetic wounds or in cases where multiple species coexists. Diabetic wounds which are polymicrobial or have complex bacterial mixtures, it becomes technically problematic to isolate and detect more than three to six species, because of varied concentrations of various species and interspecies competition (Sharma et al., 2006). Molecular techniques can also define patterns of genetic and protein expression under different clinical and morphological conditions (Price et al., 2009). Molecular approaches make possible the detection of microbes without the time required for growth and environmental selection pressures inherent in the culturing process. Although genomic tools are new in the determination of signature of microbial diversity more information is required for accurate and actionable analysis.

2.11. Inflammatory Markers and Diabetic Foot Ulcers:

The assessment and treatment of patients with chronic venous ulceration remains a massive clinical and economic burden for health care provider (Gohel et al., 2008). Low-grade immune activation represents a vital risk factor not only for the development of DM but also for several macro vascular and micro vascular complications. In diabetes the status of the immune system may be relevant at several stages in the development of chronic non-healing wounds. One of the most important of these signals is a class of molecules called cytokines. Cytokines can be generally classified as pro-inflammatory or anti-inflammatory and allow an organism to respond rapidly to an immune challenge by coordinating an appropriate immune response (Guest et al., 2008). Numerous researchers have speculated that further assessment of these factors may yield important clues regarding failed wound healing and indeed may indicate specific growth factor changes (Gohel et al., 2008).

Healing of wounds is one of the most multifaceted biological events after birth as a result of the interaction of diverse tissue structures and a large number of local and infiltrating cell types (Serra et al., 2017). The latter are mostly constituted by leukocyte subsets (macrophages, neutrophils, lymphocytes and mast cells), which in sequence infiltrate the wound location and serve as immunological effector cells and a source of inflammatory and growth-promoting cytokines (Barrientos: 2008). Because pro- and anti-inflammatory steps are crucial in the different stages of wound healing, it is possible that turbulences of the immune system interfere with tissue homeostasis and wound healing after the occurrence of ulcers and lead to the chronic, non-healing wounds that are major attribute of diabetic foot complications. Plasma levels of cytokines such as TNF-α and interleukin-6 (IL-6) were significantly raised in diabetic foot subjects when compared with diabetics without foot ulcers. Inflammatory markers such as IL-1, TNF-α have been shown to be present in significantly higher levels in chronic venous ulcers than in acute healing wounds (Beidler et al., 2009). Unfortunately, no accord exists for the optimum sampling or measuring these cytokines, and the enormous heterogeneity of cytokine levels has limited the benefit of previous research. Nevertheless, better understanding of immune mediators like cytokine and chemokine dysfunction in DFUs may inspire new therapeutic pathways. The present study also aimed to test the hypothesis that whether cytokine and chemokine concentrations relates to wound healing in patients with DFUs.

2.12. Treatment and Management of Diabetic Foot Infection:

Infected DFUs should be treated only by those with ample experience and amenities. Management of ulcers falls into three parts: subtraction of callus, abolition of infection, and lessening of weight bearing forces, often requiring bed rest with the foot raised. Excess keratin should be carefully removed with a scalpel blade to depict the floor of the ulcer and allow efficient drainage of the lesion (Jones., 1998). Virtually all clinically infected diabetic lesions require antibiotic therapy; wounds which are clinically not infected should be avoided for antibiotic treatment (Lipsky et al., 2016). Proper management requires good glycemic control with insulin, appropriate wound care and prescribed antimicrobial. The initial antibiotic therapy must usually be chosen empirically, can be modified later on the basis of availability of added clinical and microbiological results (Lipsky et al., 2015).

Prompt initiation of empirical therapy is based on chronicity of infection, available culture reports or local prevalence of pathogens especially drug resistant species. Antibiotic regime for subjects with no prior treatment with antibiotic or with mild to moderate infection should be narrow spectrum and target gram-positive cocci by oral route. The treatment of severe or more extensive infection requires broad spectrum regime targeting gram-positive cocci, obligate anaerobes and aggressive gram-negative aerobes to ensure appropriate protection (Lipsky et al., 2012).

For such infections, it is clinically recommended to start with parenteral therapy, which can be later on shifted to oral treatment when the patient is systemically well (Marvaso et al., 2002). Prior long-term or inappropriate use of antibiotics, history of hospitalization, and presence of persistent wound increases the risk of MRSA causing delayed wound healing, longer hospital stay and need of surgical interventions. Therefore, DFI harbored by MRSA should be empirically treated with an antibiotic regimen that covers MRSA (Lipsky et al., 2015). Gangrenous and stinking wounds may need anti-anaerobic treatment. Malfunctioning in treating an infected DFU with antimicrobial drugs usually associated with progressive tissue damage and sluggish wound healing. However, antibiotic therapy is linked with frequent unfavorable consequences, financial costs, and increased risk of drug resistance (Lipsky et al., 2004), so it should be reserved for treating wounds that are infected. Extent of antibiotic therapy for a DFI should be based on the chronicity of the infection, the presence or absence of infected bone and clinical response to therapy. Optimal duration of antibiotic therapy is defined on the basis of clinical studies. Records from aforementioned clinical trials reveal that most patients with just skin and soft tissue infections do well with 1–2 weeks of treatment (Lispky et al., 2015). In general, moderate and severe DFI are typically treated from 2 to 4 weeks of intravenous (IV) antibiotic therapy with 46 weeks of therapy for bone infection. Routinely advising antibiotics for a fixed period may result in an inadequate or, more often, needlessly protracted course of therapy. Antibiotics can typically be terminated once the clinical signs and symptoms of infection have rectified. There is no good verification to sustain continuing antibiotic therapy until the wound is healed in order to either speed up closure or prevent ensuing infection (Lipsky et al., 2015).

Surgical procedures are needed to drain the pus and abscess cavities and to remove all necrotic and infected tissue including devitalized and infected bone resulting from Osteomyelitis (Gibbons and Eliopoulos., 1984). Surgical interventions in treating DFIs may range from minor debridement or drainage to extensive resections in dry eschar or ischemic foot, revascularization or major amputation in non-viable limb which life threatening (e.g., necrotizing fasciitis or gas gangrene) or functionally futile. Patients with evident peripheral ischemia need revascularization as sufficient arterial blood supply is required to ease wound healing and resolve the underlying infection. Early surgical measures reduces the duration of antibiotic therapy, decreases the needs for major amputation and helps in restoration of complete ambulation (Tan et al., 1996). Delayed or inadequate surgery may impair control of infection leading to additional bone or soft tissue necrosis. On time and adequate surgical debridement, including resections or minor amputations, may decrease the likelihood of extensive amputation (Tan et al., 1996). It is advantageous to preserve as much distal viable soft tissue and bone as possible during amputation, potentially allowing for late closure and efficient weight bearing. Skin grafting is seldom needed and accelerates wound healing. Heterogeneous feature of diabetic wounds requires dressing selection on the basis of location, size, depth and amount of necrotic tissue. Dry necrotic tissue should be dressed continuously with moistened saline gauze whereas for necrotic lesions hydrogels are preferred. Foam dressings wick up and lock in large volumes of exudates (Hinchliffee et al., 2008). Careful monitoring of the wound is requisite with any dressing practice. Use of a total contact plaster cast, light-weight scotch cast boot, or air cast boots may aid healing. These conform to the contours of the foot, thereby dipping shear forces on the plantar aspect. Casts should be removed every week for wound inspection and then renewed. Once the ulcer is healed, the patient should be assessed for cradled insoles and bespoke shoes. Diabetic patients, who adhere to routine foot care, with daily self-exam of the feet and podiatry care, are less prone to develop ulcers than those who don't follow foot care recommendations (Papanas et al., 2012). However, many patients fail to sustain self-care procedures over time. Studies have evaluated that less than one-third of patients with diabetes and active foot ulcers regularly wear recommended offloading devices during activities (Dorresteijn et al., 2012).

Patients suffering from foot ulcers experience poor quality of life due to sedentary lifestyle, social isolation, hindrances in work and leisure activities, depression, and pain. Therefore clinicians or nurses routinely assessing patients with diabetes for foot ulcers can ensure that ulcers are examined at earliest and treated appropriately to reduce complications and improve patient's quality of life (Bengtsson et al., 2008.

Materials and Methods

3. MATERIALS AND METHODS

3.1. Study Design:

This was a prospective cohort hospital based study. Ninety type 2 diabetic patients suffering from DFUs (Wagners Grade 0-IV), admitted in endocrinology ward of Rajiv Gandhi Centre for Diabetes and Endocrinology, Jawaharlal Nehru Medical College, Aligarh Muslim University, Aligarh, India, during May 2014 to April 2016 were enrolled in the study. The informed consent was given by all subjects and the study was approved by and Bio-Ethical Committee (BEC) of Faculty of Medicine, Jawaharlal Nehru Medical College, Aligarh Muslim University, Aligarh.

The enrolled subjects were diagnosed DM according to guidelines of ADA- 2014.

- Fasting plasma glucose ≥126 mg/dL (7.0 mmol/L). Fasting is defined as no calorie intake for 8 hours. OR
- Post prandial plasma glucose ≥200 mg/dL (11. 0 mmol/L) during an Oral Glucose Tolerance Test (OGTT). The test was performed as defined by World Health Organization, using a glucose load containing 75 gm anhydrous glucose dissolved in water. OR
- Presence of classical symptoms of hyperglycemia with random plasma glucose ≥200 mg/dL (11.1mmol/L).

3.2. Clinical Analysis:

On the day of admission, a detailed history and physical examination was done of every subject. Patients were evaluated for age, sex, duration of diabetes, BMI, glycemic status, lipid profile. Furthermore, subjects were also assessed for secondary complications such as retinopathy and its stage (Within normal limits, WNL; Non-proliferative diabetic retinopathy, NPDR; Pre-proliferative Diabetic retinopathy, PPDR; Proliferative Diabetic Retinopathy, PDR; according to International Clinical Diabetic Retinopathy Disease Severity Scale (Klein et al., 1998). Neuropathy was assessed on the absence of perception of the Semmes-Weinstein monofilament at 2 of 10 defined plantar sites on either foot (Mayfield et al., 2000), PVD on ischemic symptoms or absence of posterior or tibial pedal pulses. Ankle brachial Index (ABI) was calculated by ratio of ankle systolic blood pressure (defined as higher of the dorsal pedis or posterior tibial artery) and higher brachial pressure. Subjects were diagnosed for PVD when ankle brachial index (ABI) ≤ 0.9 or they had undergone a peripheral arterial bypass or previous amputation (Weitz et al., 1996). Nephropathy was defined and staged according to estimated glomerular filtration rate (eGFR) (Stage 1, eGFR$\geq$90 mL/min/1.73m^2; Stage 2, eGFR 60-89 mL/min/1.73 m^2; Stage 3, eGFR 30-59 mL/min/1.73 m^2; Stage 4, eGFR 15-29 mL/min/1.73 m^2; Stage 5, eGFR <15 mL/min/1.73 m^2) (Levey et al., 2009).

The enrolled subjects were defined hypertensive according to ADA criteria, systolic blood pressure $\geq$140 mmHg or diastolic blood pressure $\geq$90 mmHg or on antihypertensive treatment during the time of admission. Serum cholesterol levels $\geq$ 150 mg/dL and triglycerides $\geq$200 mg/dL, serum LDL- cholesterol > 100 mg/dL, HDL-cholesterol <40 mg/dL (for males) and < 50 mg/dL for females were used to define diabetic dyslipidemia (Sehri et al., 2014). Coronary artery disease (CAD) was defined on the basis of history of physician diagnosed angina, myocardial infarction, or any previous revascularization procedure as determined during questionnaire (Sehri et al., 2014). CVD was assessed by history or specific neurological examination done by specialist, and hospitalized or radiological (brain computed tomography or brain magnetic resonance) records of transient ischemic attack (TIA) or stroke (Sehri et al., 2014). All clinical investigations including serum creatinine, urine micro-albumin, lipid profile, fasting and post prandial blood glucose, HbA1c, hemogram were done on the day of admission.

3.3. Foot Analysis:

The ulcer of foot was analyzed clinically, encompassing location, duration of ulcer, size of ulcer, pre-ulcerations and history of amputation. The size of ulcer was calculated by multiplying the longest and widest section and expressed as centimeter square. Infection was clinically defined by presence of edema, erythema, purulent discharge, and cellulitis and tissue necrosis (Lispky et al., 2012). The lesions were graded according to Wagner's classification system at the time of hospitalization.

Grade 0 (no open lesion), grade I (superficial ulcer), grade II (deep ulcer upto tendons and joint tissue), grade III (deep ulcer with abscess, osteomyelitis, and joint sepsis), grade IV (local gangrene forefoot or heel) and grade V (gangrene of entire foot figure 10). Patients with grade 0 were excluded from the study. Diagnosis of bone infection was made by probing with sterile steel probe or plain radiographs. Amputation was defined as loss of any part of lower extremity in the transverse anatomical plane (Hartemann Heurtier 2004).

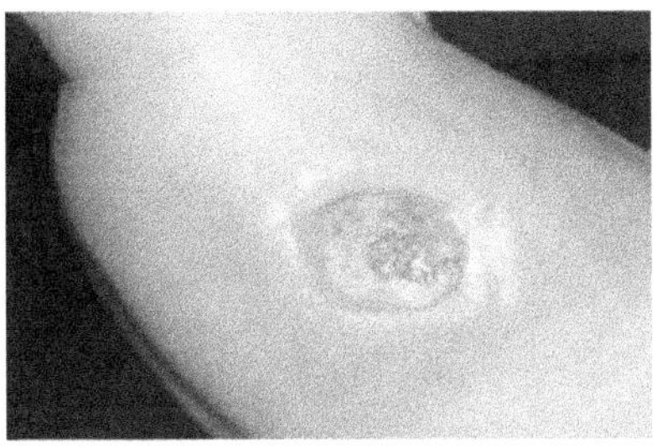

Grade I: Superficial Ulcer

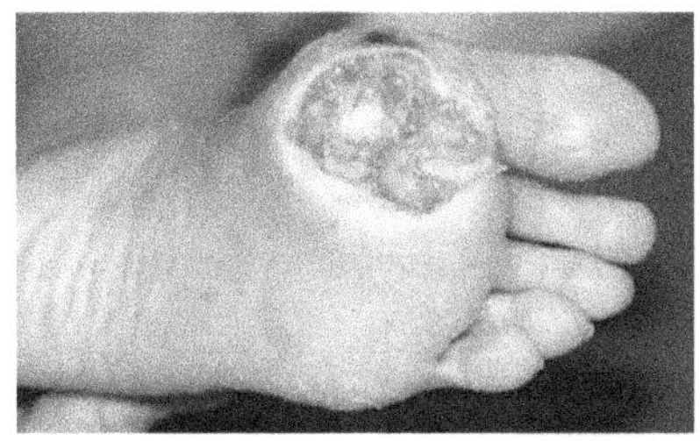

Grade II: Ulcer upto tendon/capsule

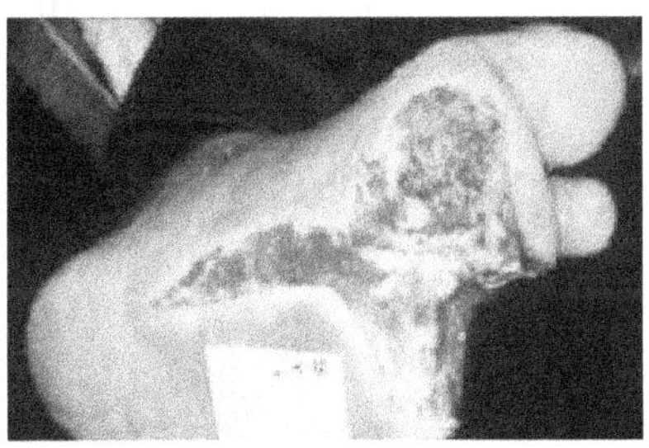

Grade III: Ulcer penetrating the bones

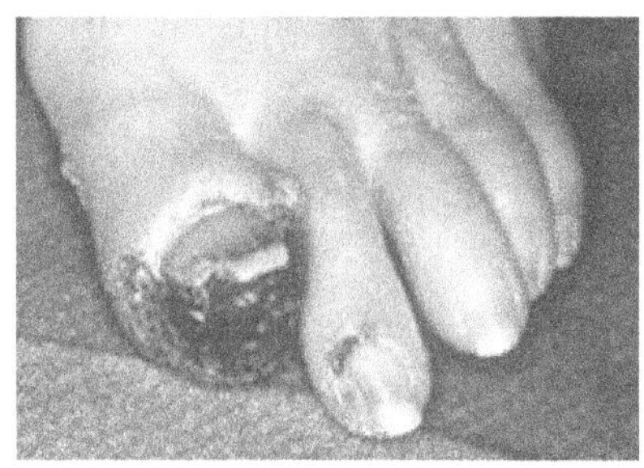

Grade IV: Partial Gangrene

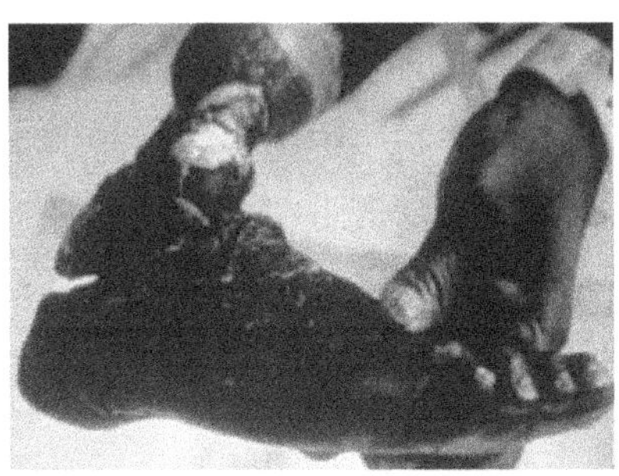

Grade V: Gangrene of complete foot

Figure 10: Wagner's Grading for Diabetic Foot Ulcers

3.4. Biochemical Investigations:

3.4.1. Sample collection:

Venous blood samples were collected after an overnight fasting, and centrifuged at 3000 rpm for 5 min at 4 degree. Serum/ plasma was separated and stored at –80 ^{0}C till further analysis. Blood samples were collected in:

- In ethylenediaminetetraacetic acid (EDTA) vials for HbA1c
- In sodium fluoride vials for plasma glucose
- In plain vials for serum lipids and lipoproteins

3.4.2. Plasma Glucose estimation:

Principle: Glucose oxidase catalyzes the oxidation of alpha- D- glucose to D-glucono-1, 5 lactone with the formation of hydrogen peroxides. The lactone is then slowly hydrolysed to D-gluconic acid. The hydrogen peroxide produced is then broken down to oxygen and water by a peroxidase enzyme. Oxygen then react with an oxygen acceptor such as ortho toluidine which itself converted to a coloured compound, the amount of which can be measured colorimetrically. Estimation of plasma glucose by this method eliminates the interference by other reducing sugars (McMilin et al., 1990).

3.4.3. Glycated Hemoglobin estimation:

Principle: The D-10 Hemoglobin A1c Program utilizes principles of ion-exchange high-performance liquid chromatography (HPLC). The samples are automatically diluted on the D-10 and injected into the analytical cartridge. The D-10 delivers a programmed buffer gradient of increasing ionic strength to the cartridge, where the hemoglobins are separated based on their ionic interactions with the cartridge material. The separated hemoglobins then pass through the flow cell of the filter photometer, where changes in the absorbance at 415 nm are measured. The assay procedures were followed as per directives of the kit, Bio- Rad Laboratories Inc., Hercules, California, USA.

3.4.4. Serum Lipids estimation:

3.4.4.1. Serum Cholesterol:

Total serum cholesterol was estimated by method of cholesterol oxidase per-oxidase method purchased from Avantor Performance material India Limited Dehradun, Uttarakhand, India. The intensity of colour produced during the set of reactions at 520 nm is directly proportional to the concentration of total cholesterol.

3.4.4.2. Serum Triglycerides:

TAGs were estimated by method Glycerol Phosphatase Oxidase and Peroxidase (Liquid Stable) purchased from Avantor Performance Material India, Limited, Dehradun, Uttarakhand, India. The estimations were conducted according to the instructions provided in the kit manual.

3.4.4.3. HDL- Cholesterol:

After centrifugation, HDL remains in the supernatant. The serum cholesterol in the HDL fraction is estimated by using the method polyethylene glycol (PEG) and phenol and 4-aminoantipyrine (PAP) purchased from Avantor Performance Material India, Limited, Dehradun, Uttarakhand, India.

3.4.4.4. LDL- Cholesterol:

Principle: The estimation of LDL- cholesterol was done using Freidwald and Fredrickson formula (Roberts., 1988)

LDL-cholesterol= Total Cholesterol-(Triglycerides/5 + HDL- C)

3.5. Conventional Microbiological Analysis:

3.5.1. Collection of pus/ tissue samples for aerobic bacteria:

Ninety diabetic foot subjects were admitted, out of which 20 subjects with ulcers of Grade 0 were excluded from the study. The samples for aerobic culture were obtained on the day of admission from 70 type 2 diabetic subjects with infected DFUs. The ulcer was vigorously washed with normal saline and debrided to remove exudates. The base of ulcer was scraped by rolling a sterile transport swab with Amies media without charcoal purchased from HiMedia (Product number MS684-50No, HiMedia Mumbai, India). The samples were immediately processed within 20 minutes for identification of pathogens (Gadepalli et al., 2006).

3.5.2. Sample Processing:

3.5.2.1. Direct microscopy:

The smears were made from the pus specimens obtained from DFUs to identify the presence of gram-positive and gram-negative cocci/bacilli. The smears on the sterile slides were heat fixed to adhere the smear on slide. The smears were gently stained with cystal violet solution followed by Grams iodine. The smears of killed bacteria were decolorized using 95% ethyl alcohol. The slides after rinsing with distilled water and counter stained with safranin were viewed under light microscope (Patrick., 2007).

3.5.2.2. Culture and Identification of Aerobic Isolates

The pus samples were inoculated on the, Teepol Lactose Agar, blood agar plate (BA), nutrient agar (NA) and simultaneously brain heart infusion (BHI) broth and incubated at 37 ^{o} C for 18 hrs (CLSI). The aerobic isolates were identified according to morphology, culture characteristics, metabolism and biochemical properties (Wayne; 2008).

3.5.3. Antimicrobial Susceptibility Testing:

Antimicrobial susceptibility testing was done for aerobic bacteria by Kirby Bauer disk diffusion method on Mueller Hilton agar (MHA) plates according to Clinical and Laboratory Standards Institute (CLSI) guidelines (Wayne., 2006). Commercially prepared antimicrobial discs were obtained from HiMedia Laboratories Mumbai, India. Following antimicrobials were used piperacillin (100 μg), aztreonam (30 μg), cefepime (30 μg), amikacin (30 μg), cefeperazone (75 μg), piperacillin/tazobactum (100/10 μg), cefeperazone/sulbactum (75/10 μg), cefexime (5 ug), ofloxacin (5 μg), ceftazidime/clavulanic acid (30/10 μg), ceftazidime (30 μg), levofloxacin (5 μg), clindamycin (2 μg), vancomycin (30 μg), tobramycin (10 μg), Erythromycin (25 μg), Sparfloxacin (5 μg). MRSA were determined by using 1 μg oxacillin disc (NCCLS 2002). These drugs were stored in cartridges long with desiccant at -20 °C in freezer. A small working supple of disc was also kept at 4 °C maximum of one week. On removal from refrigerator for usage, the containers were kept at room temperature for one hour. This allowed the disc to equilibrate at room temperature thus minimizing the amount of condensation that occurs when warm air comes in contact with cold discs.

*3.5.3.1. **Procedures:***

Sterile disposable petri plates were poured with 25- 30 ml autoclaved MHA media with a uniform depth of 4 mm. These plates were stored at 4 °C until use. The test strains were grown overnight, and few colonies were picked up and suspended into sterile nutrient containing broth. Within fifteen minutes of inoculation, a sterile swab was dipped into the test inoculums and streaked over the surface medium three times by rotating the plate at 60 degree after each application. The streaked petri plates were dried at room temperature with closed lids. Antibiotic discs were then placed on the surface of dried petri plates with sterile forceps and gently pressed down to ensure proper and even contact of medium with disc. Plates were incubated at 37 °C for 18 hrs.

*3.5.3.2. **Interpretation:***

Diameter of zone and disk was measured with the help of zone scale in mm. The plate was illuminated with reflected light at 45 degree angle by placing at 3 inches above a black background. End point of inhibition was judged by naked eye to the point of abrupt diminution of growth or to the point of 80% inhibition as per the recommendation of CLSI-2007. *Staphylococcus* species resistant to 1 μg of oxacillin disk and 30 μg of cefoxitin were considered as MRSA positive (Wayne., 2006).

3.6. Molecular Methods for Bacterial Identification:

The genotypic identification of bacterial flora harboring the wound was done using polymerase chain reaction. The genotypic protocol involves

- Isolation of DNA from specimens obtained from infected ulcers
- PCR for identification of most common pathogens prevalent in northern India
- Agarose gel electrophoresis.

3.6.1. Isolation of DNA:

The pus samples collected from wounds of 70 type 2 diabetic subjects with infected DFUs after washing vigorously with normal saline and proper debridement, were suspended in sterile test tubes containing nutrient broth. The inoculums were allowed to grow overnight in incubation at 37 ^{0}C. The samples were processed next day for isolation of DNA using GenElute ^{TM} Bacterial Genomic DNA kit (Sigma Aldrich). The pellet from 1.5 ml of overnight bacteria was formed by centrifuging at 12000-16000 x g for 2 min. The pellet was resuspended in 180 μl of Lysis solution T and RNase was added to remove any RNA content. The sample processed was then added with 20 μl of proteinase K to bring protein lysis followed by addition of Lysis solution C. This method combines the advantage of silica based system with microspin format. The bacteria are lysed in a chaotropic salt containing solution to ensure the thorough denaturation of macromolecules. The addition of ethanol causes DNA to bind when the cell lysate is spun through a silica membrane into a micro-centrifuge tube. After washing with washing solution to remove contaminants the DNA is eluted in 200 μl of Tris-EDTA solution.

The eluted DNA was immediately stored at -20^{0}C until processed.

3.6.2. PCR Amplification:

The DNA samples were processed for identification of microbial etiology by using species specific primers for the most common isolates prevalent in DFI in northern India. The organisms targeted in the study were:

1. ***Staphylococcus aureus***
2. ***Klebsiella species***
3. ***Pseudomonas aeruginosa***
4. ***Escherichia coli***

Following list of primers were used for identification of the above mentioned pathogens.

Table 10: PCR primers used in the study

Microorganisms	Primer sequences	Tm (^{0}C)	Product size (bps)	Reference
Staphylococcus aureus	F-GATTGATGGTGATACGGT	57	273	(Melendez et al., 2010)
	R- CAAGCCTTGACGAACTA			
Klebsiella species	F-CAACGGTGTGGTTACTGACG	55	108	(Chander et al., 2011)
	R-TCTACGAAGTGGCCGTTTTC			
Pseudomonas aeruginosa	F-GGGGGATCTTCGGACCTCA	58	956	(Coenye et al., 2002)
	R-TCCTTAGAGTGCCCACCCG			
Escherichia coli	F-CCGATACGCTGCCAATCAGT	55	884	(Chen et al., 1998)
	R-ACGCAGACCGTAGGCCAGAT			

bps, basepairs, **F**, forward; **R**, reverse

3.6.3. Reaction Mixture and Cycling Conditions:

A] Detection of *Klebsiella species*

Preparation of reaction mixture

The reaction mixture for PCR was prepared using the following reagents in given amount and sequence.

Table 11: Reagents used in preparation of reaction mixture

Reagent	Quantity for 50 µl of reaction mixture
Forward Primer (mM)	0.1 µl
Reverse Primer (mM)	0.1 µl
2X Mater Mix	25 µl
Template DNA solution (200 ng)	5 µl
Nuclease water	19.8 µl

Cycling conditions for identification of Klebsiella species

PCR was carried out in thermal cycler with a first cycle of denaturation at 94 °C for 7 min, then 35 cycles of denaturation at 94 °C for 50 sec, annealing at 55 °C for 50 sec, and elongation at 72 °C for 1 min 30 sec. The PCR was completed by final elongation at 72 °C for 10 mins.

B] Detection of *Pseudomonas aeruginosa*

Preparation of reaction mixture

The reaction mixture for PCR was prepared using the following reagents in given amount and sequence.

Table 12: Reagents used in preparation of reaction mixture

Reagent	Quantity for 50 µl of reaction mixture
Forward Primer	0.1 µl (mM)
Reverse Primer	0.1 µl (mM)
2X Mater Mix	25 µl
Template DNA solution	5 µl (200 ng)
Nuclease water	19.8 µl

Cycling conditions for identification of Pseudomonas aeruginosa

PCR was carried out in thermal cycler with a first cycle of denaturation at 95 °C for 15 min, then 30 cycles of denaturation at 94 °C for 1 min, annealing at 58 °C for 2 mins and elongation at 74 °C for 3 min. The PCR was completed by final elongation at 72 °C for 10 mins.

C] Detection of *Escherichia coli*

Preparation of reaction mixture

The reaction mixture for PCR was prepared using the following reagents in given amount and sequence.

Table 13: Reagents used in preparation of reaction mixture

Reagent	Quantity for 50 µl of reaction mixture
Forward Primer (mM)	0.1 µl
Reverse Primer (mM)	0.1 µl
2X Mater Mix	25 µl
Template DNA solution (200 ng)	5 µl
Nuclease water	19.8 µl

Cycling conditions for identification of Escherichia coli

PCR was carried out in thermal cycler with a first cycle of denaturation at 94 °C for 10 min, then 30 cycles of denaturation at 95 °C for 1 min, annealing at 55 °C for 2 min and elongation at 72 °C for 10 min. The PCR was completed by final elongation at 72 °C for 10 mins.

D] Detection of Staphylococcus aureus

Preparation of reaction mixture

The reaction mixture for PCR was prepared using the following reagents in given amount and sequence.

Table 14: Reagents used in preparation of reaction mixture

Reagent	**Quantity for 50 μl of reaction mixture**
Forward Primer (mM)	0.1 μl
Reverse Primer (mM)	0.1 μl
2X Mater Mix	25 μl
Template DNA solution (200 ng)	5 μl
Nuclease water	19.8 μl

Cycling conditions for identification of Staphylococcus aureus

PCR was carried out in thermal cycler with a first cycle of denaturation at 94^0C for 10 mins, then 30 cycles of denaturation at 95^0C for 1 min, annealing at 57^0C for 60 sec and elongation at 72 ^{0}C for 10 min. The PCR was completed by final elongation at 72 ^{o}C for 10 min.

3.6.4. TAE Buffer Preparation:

Table 15: Following reagents were used in preparation of TAE buffer

Reagents	**Quantity**
Tris base	242 gms
Glacial Acetic acid	57.1 ml
0.5 M Disodium EDTA (pH 8)	100 ml
Double distilled water	1000 ml

3.6.5. Agarose Gel Electrophoresis:

3.6.5.1. Principle

Gel electrophoresis is a technique which is use to separate a mixture of molecules of various sizes and shape by passing them through a stationary material (gel) under electric field. Wells were prepared in gel using comb of appropriate size. The sample containing DNA of various sizes were loaded in each well and allowed to sieve through the gel under electric field. As the separation process continues, smaller DNA molecules move faster than larger ones. Molecular weight markers were also loaded to determine the size of fragments in the sample DNA.

3.6.5.2. Preparation of Agarose gel

The agarose gel was prepared by boiling molecular grade agarose (Sigma Aldrich India) in 0.5 X TAE buffer to dissolve it completely. After cooling it to about 50 degree Celsius, 1 ul (0.5 μg/mL) solution of ethidium bromide dye (Sigma Aldrich, India) was added. Before dissolving the agarose, the casting platform was placed on a leveled surface with the help of gel caster. The comb was then placed across the gel-casting platform, so that the teeth of the comb remained 1 mm above the base of platform. The molten agarose was then slowly poured on to the gel casting platform and it was kept undisturbed for about an hour to solidify the gel. After the gel solidifies, the comb was taken out and tray was removed from the caster. The set gel along with caster was submerged in the electrophoresis tank (Biorad+, India) with the wells at the cathode end of the tank with sufficient quantity (above 1mm level) of 1 X TAE buffer.

PCR product (10 ul) was mixed with 6X bromo-phenol blue loading dye (2 ul) and was loaded carefully in the respective wells. First or last well was used for loading standard molecular weight markers (1000 bp) purchased from Thermo scientific. Electrophoresis was done at 6 V/cm and the progress of mobility was monitored by visualizing the migration of dye. After completion of electrophoresis, the gel was removed and visualized under Gel Documentation system (BioRad, Germany) for the bands of desired molecular weight.

3.7. Estimation of Cytokine Levels:

Pro- and anti-inflammatory cytokines were estimated in the serum/plasma samples of diabetic foot patients using commercially available enzyme linked immune-sorbent assay (ELISA) kits. The human cytokine array kit was purchased from R&D System, Canada, USA. All assays were performed according to manufacturer's instructions.

Generally in regular ELISA kits, antibody specific for the cytokine of interest is bound to the walls of plastic microtiter wells. Samples are incubated in the wells, and any cytokine in the sample gets bound to the antibody on the well walls. The wells are then washed, and a second antibody (Horseradish peroxidase (HRP)- conjugated antibody) is added to this one also specific for the cytokine, but recognizing epitopes different from those bound by the first antibody. After incubation, the wells are washed again, removing any unattached antibody. Attached to the second antibody is an enzyme, which, when presented with its substrate (Tetramethylbenzidine (TMB), produces a colored product, the intensity of the color produced being proportional to the amount of bound cytokine. The intensity of the color is then read by a spectrophotometer at 450 nm wave length. In high sensitivity kits a biotin-conjugated antibody is added first followed by streptavidin-HRP antibody after washing. Then, two amplification reagents are added, namely biotinyl-tyramide and streptavidin-HRP, separated by a washing step. This is followed by the TMB substrate solution. The intensity of the color is then read by a spectrophotometer at 450 nm. To find the difference in the level of inflammatory markers, serum/plasma from 40 type 2 diabetic subjects (control group) without foot ulcers was also collected.

3.8. Statistical Analysis:

The base line data was analyzed using SPSS version 17.0 for descriptive statistics. Quantitative variables were expressed as means ± SD while qualitative variables as percentages (%). Continuous variables between the groups were compared with student t test and categorical variables by Chi square test. A Pearson co-relation analysis and multiple regression analysis were used to assess the association between all the variables. A two tailed p value (<0.05) was considered as statistically significant.

Results

4. RESULTS

4.1. Clinical and Demographical Variables of Diabetic Foot Subjects:

The demographical profile and clinical variables of 70 patients with infected DFU are listed in Table 17 (Grade I-IV). In this study males were predominant 51 (49.3%) as compared to females 19 (27.1%). The age ≥ 41 years predominated. The majority of patients, 31 (44.2%) had diabetes more than 10 years. Twenty five (35.7%) were overweight (BMI, 23.0-24.9 kg/m^2) and 20 (28.5%) were obese (BMI > 25 kg/m^2) and rest were lean (BMI< 18.5 kg/m^2). Five (7.14%) subjects had good glycemic control with HbA1c <6.5% on the admission day, 65 (92.8%), had poor glycemic state with HbA1c ≥ 6.5%. HDL-cholesterol (< 40 mg/dL), was found in 49 (70%) patients, TAGs (> 200 mg/dL) in 44 (62.8%), and LDL-cholesterol (>100 mg/dL) was observed in 64 (91.4%). Nearly two third, 55 (78.5%) had ulcer of ≥ 1 month and majority, 30 (42.8%) had size of ulcer ≥ 4 cm^2. Among the subjects enrolled those with grade II and IV predominated, 24 (34.2%) each. Nineteen (27.1%) subjects had ulcers of grade III and 3 (4.2%) subjects had grade I ulcers. Twenty nine (41.4%) patients were diagnosed hypertensive (BP ≥ 140/90 mmHg or on anti-hypertensive drug, 28 (40%) had peripheral neuropathy, 56 (80%) had nephropathy, 49 (70%) retinopathy and 44 (62.8%) had PVD. Forty three (61.4%) subjects were diagnosed for osteomyelitis. Majority of subjects 30 (42.8%), underwent minor amputation and 3 (4.2%) received major amputation. Female patients had higher prevalence of ulcer size ≥ 4cm^2 than males. In this study male patients had higher prevalence of secondary complications including retinopathy, nephropathy, PVD and osteomyelitis than females.

Table 16: Clinical and demographical variables of 70 subjects with DFU

Characteristics	Total	Male	Female	*p* value
n	70	51	19	
Age (yrs)				
21-40	13	10 (19.6%)	3 (15.7%)	NS
41-70	57	41 (80.3%)	16 (84.2%)	-------
Diabetes duration (yrs)				
<10	39	28 (54.9%)	11 (57.8%)	NS
≥10	31	23 (45.0%)	8 (15.6%)	
BMI (kg/m^2)				
Lean (<18.5)	8	6 (11.7%)	2 (10.5%)	NS
Normal (18.5-22.9)	17	12 (23.5%)	5 (26.3%)	NS
Overweight (23.0-24.9)	25	19 (37.2%)	6 (31.5%)	NS
Obese (≥25)	20	14 (27.4%)	6 (31.5%)	NS
HbA1c (%)				
<6.5	5	5 (9.8%)	0 (0.0%)	NS
≥6.5	65	46 (90.1%)	19 (100%)	--------
Lipid Analysis				
Se TC >150 mg/dL	51	35 (68.6%)	16 (84.2%)	NS
Se TAG>200 mg/dL	44	35 (68.6%)	9 (47.3%)	NS
Se HDL-C < 40 mg/dL	49	38 (74.5%)	11 (57.8%)	**<0.01**
Se LDL-C >100 mg/dL	52	41 (80.3%)	11 (57.8%)	NS
Size of ulcer				
<4 cm^2	25	20 (39.2%)	5 (26.3%)	-------
≥ 4cm^2	45	30 (58.8%)	15 (78.9%)	**<0.05**
Ulcer duration				
<1 month	15	10 (19.6%)	5 (26.3%)	NS
≥1 month	55	41 (80.3%)	14 (73.6%)	-------
Grade of ulcer				
I	3	2 (3.9%)	1 (5.2%)	NS
II	24	21 (41.1%)	3 (15.7%)	NS
III	19	11 (21.5%)	8 (42.1%)	NS
IV	24	17 (33.3%)	7 (36.8%)	NS
Complications				
Hypertension	29	20 (39.2%)	9 (47.3%)	NS
Retinopathy	49	43 (84.3%)	6 (31.5%)	**<0.001**
Neuropathy	28	21 (41.1%)	7 (36.8%)	NS
Nephropathy	56	49 (96.0%)	7 (36.9%)	**<0.001**
Peripheral vascular disease	44	38 (74.5%)	6 (31.5%)	**<0.01**
Osteomyelitis	43	37 (72.5%)	6 (31.5%)	**<0.01**
Amputation				
Minor	30	22 (43.1%)	8 (42.1%)	NS
Major	3	3 (5.8%)	0 (0.0%)	--------

n, number of patients; **BMI**, body mass index; **HbA1c**: glycated hemoglobin; **Se TC**, serum total cholesterol; **Se TAG**, serum triglycerides; **Se HDL-C**, serum high density lipoprotein-cholesterol; **Se LDL-C**, serum low-density lipoprotein-cholesterol; **NS**, not significant.

4.2. Baseline Characteristics of Diabetic Foot Subjects with Healing and Non-Healing Ulcers:

4.2.1. Demographical Variables:

Out of ninety type 2 diabetic patients with DFUs admitted to endocrinology ward, seventy had clinically infected DFUs. Patients were grouped depending upon healing and non-healing state of ulcer following routine examination based on healing signs/symptoms. Routine clinical examination of ulcers was done up-to two months from the day of admission to evaluate the healing status. Non-healing lesions were clinically diagnosed on the basis of absence of epithelialization, angiogenesis, and formation of granulation tissues. Patients with non-healing wounds were significantly older than those without it ($p < 0.05$). HbA1c ($p < 0.05$), fasting plasma glucose ($p < 0.05$), serum TAG ($p < 0.01$) and LDL-C ($p < 0.01$) were significantly elevated in subjects with non-healed ulcers as compared to those without it. Patients with non-healing infected ulcers had had a higher prevalence of neuropathy ($p < 0.05$), PVD ($p < 0.05$) and osteomyelitis ($p < 0.05$) than those with healing ulcers. Surgical amputations of lower limb were significantly higher in subjects with non-healing wounds ($p < 0.05$) (Table 18).

4.2.2. Ulcer Characteristics:

Among the subjects, the mean duration of infected ulcer was 1.45 ± 0.6 months. Size of ulcer ≥ 4 cm^2 was observed in 45 (64.3%) cases and < 4 cm^2 in 25 (35.7%) subjects. Surgical amputation was done in 33 (47.1%) subjects, of which 3 (4.3%) underwent major amputation, and 30 (42.8%) were subjected to minor amputation. Diabetic foot wounds of non-healing category were significantly long-standing than healing wounds ($p < 0.05$). Of total seventy subjects, 19 (27.1%) were on antibiotics before admission, 10 (14.3%) were unaware of previous medication whereas rest of the subjects did not receive antibiotics. Seventy percent patients had no prior knowledge of diabetes linked secondary complications and foot care (Table 18).

Table 17: Characteristics of Diabetic Foot Subjects with Healing and Non-Healing Ulcers

Characteristics	Healing Ulcers	Non-Healing Ulcers	*p* value
n	27	43	
Male (%)	22 (78.5%)	29 (82.5%)	NS
Age (yrs)	50.2 ± 10.8	55.9 ± 11.6	**<0.05**
Diabetes duration (yrs)	7.6 ± 5.5	7.4 ± 5.1	NS
BMI (kg/m^2)	25.5 ± 5.2	31.1 ± 3.1	**<0.0001**
HbA1c (%)	9.1± 2.0	11 ± 3.6	**<0.05**
FPG (mg/dL)	170 ± 44.2	200.7 ± 58.6	**<0.05**
Se. Cr (mg/dL)	1.4 ± 0.8	1.2 ± 0.5	NS
Lipid profile			
Se TC (mg/dL)	164.2 ± 22.4	170.2 ± 29.43	NS
Se TAGs (mg/dL)	148.3 ± 38.9	183.1 ± 54.8	**<0.01**
Se HDL (mg/dL)	47.6 ±10.1	39.4 ± 6.6	**<0.0001**
Se LDL (mg/dL)	71.6 ± 11.3	78.0 ± 6.1	**<0.01**
Size of ulcer			
<4 cm^2	13 (48.1%)	12 (27.9%)	**<0.05**
≥ 4cm^2	14 (51.8%)	31 (72%)	
Ulcer duration (months)	1.2 ± 0.7	1.7 ± 0.6	**<0.05**
Grade of ulcer			
I	1 (3.7%)	2 (4.6%)	NS
II	11 (40.7%)	13 (30.2%)	NS
III	5 (18.5%)	12 (27.9%)	NS
IV	8 (29.6%)	16 (37.2%)	NS
Complications			
Hypertension	11 (39.2%)	18 (45.7%)	NS
Retinopathy	20 (71.4%)	29 (77.1%)	NS
Neuropathy	16 (39%)	12 (24.3%)	**<0.05**
Nephropathy	24 (85.3%)	32 (95.4%)	NS
Peripheral vascular disease	15 (53.5%)	29 (78.3%)	**<0.05**
Osteomyelitis	12 (35.7%)	31 (78.3%)	**<0.05**
Amputation	8 (29.6%)	25 (58.1%)	**<0.05**
Minor	8 (29.6%)	22 (51.1%)	NS
Major	0 (0%)	3 (6.9%)	------

n, number of patients; **BMI**, body mass index; **HbA1c**, glycated hemoglobin; **FPG**, fasting plasma glucose; **Se Cr**, serum creatinine; **Se TC**, total cholesterol; **Se TAG**, total triglycerides; **Se HDL-C**, high-density-lipoprotein-cholesterol; **Se LDL-C**, low-density lipoprotein- cholesterol; **NS**, not significant.

4.3. Analysis of Risk Factors for Non-Healing Ulcers:

In a uni-variate analysis, odds ratio (OR) and risk ratio (RR) were calculated between the two groups (healing ulcers and non-healing ulcers). Significant factors which were more likely to be associated with non-healing ulcers were, serum TAGs >200 mg/dL ($p < 0.05$; OR = 0.27; RR = 0. 59), serum HDL-C <40 mg/dL ($p < 0.01$; OR = 0.18; RR = 0.57), presence of grade III ulcer ($p < 0.05$; OR = 3.22; RR = 1.99), size of ulcer ≥ 4 cm^2 ($p < 0.01$; OR = 0.24; RR = 0.63), ulcers on heel of foot ($p < 0.01$; OR = 0.16; RR = 0.22), neuropathy (p= <0.01; OR= 3.7; RR= 2.12), and osteomyelitis (p <0.01; OR = 0.31; RR = 0.62) (Table 19).

Table 18: Risk Factors for Non-Healing Ulcers

Factors	**Healing Ulcers**	**Non-Healing Ulcers**	***p value***	**OR (95% CI)**	**RR (95% CI)**
n (%)	27 (38.5 %)	43 (61.4%)			
Sex (Male)	22 (81.4)	29 (67.4)	NS	2.12 (0.66-6.7)	1.20 (0.91-1.59)
Age (≥41 years)	19 (70.3)	38 (88.3)	NS	0.31 (0.08-1.08)	0.79 (0.60-1.04)
HbA1c (≥6.5%)	25 (92.7)	40(93.0)	NS	0.93 (0.14-6.00)	0.99 (0.87-1.13)
Lipid spectra					
Se TC >150 mg/dL	17 (62.9)	34 (79.0)	NS	0.45 (0.15-1.31)	0.79 (0.57-1.10)
Se TAG >200 mg/dL	12 (44.4)	32 (74.4)	**<0.05**	**0.27 (0.09-0.76)**	**0.59 (0.37-0.94)**
Se HDL-C <40 mg/dL	13 (48.1)	36 (83.7)	**<0.01**	0.18 (0.05-0.54)	0.57 (0.38-0.86)
Se LDL-C >100 mg/dL	21 (77.7)	31 (72.0)	NS	1.35 (0.43-4.17)	1.07 (0.82-1.41)
Grade of Ulcer					
I	1(3.7)	2 (4.6)	NS	**0.78 (0.06-9.13)**	**0.79(0.07-8.36)**
II	11 (40.7)	13 (30.2)	NS	1.57 (0.57-4.34)	1.34 (0.70-2.56)
III	15 (55.5)	12 (27.9)	**<0.05**	**3.2 (1.17-8.8)**	1.99 (0.47-1.08)
IV	8 (29.6)	16 (37.2)	NS	0.71 (0.152-1.14)	0.71(0.39-1.6)
Size of ulcer ≥4 cm^2	14 (51.8)	35 (81.3)	**<0.05**	**0.24 (0.08-0.72)**	**0.63 (0.43-0.94)**
Ulcer ≥1 month	15 (55.5)	40 (93.0)	**<0.0001**	**0.09 (0.02-0.37)**	**0.59 (0.42-0.84)**
Site of ulcer					
Interdigit	3 (11.1)	6 (13.9)	NS	0.77 (0.17-3.37)	0.79 (0.21-2.92)
Plantar	9 (33.3)	15 (34.8)	NS	0.93 (0.33-2.57)	0.95 (0.48-1.87)
Heel	2 (7.40)	14 (32.5)	**<0.05**	**0.16 (0.03-0.80)**	**0.22 (0.05-0.92)**
Margins	6 (22.2)	7 (16.2)	NS	1.46 (0.43-4.95)	1.36 (0.51-3.63)
Malleoli	3 (11.1)	3 (6.9)	NS	0.23(0.026-2.089)	0.26 (0.03-2.08)
Multiple site (>2)	4 (14.8)	0 (0)	----		----
Complications					
Hypertension	11 (39.2%)	18 (45.7%)	NS	0.95 (0.35-2.5)	0.97(0.54-1.73)
Retinopathy	20 (71.4%	29 (77.1%)	NS	1.37 (0.47-4.02)	1.09 (0.80-1.48)
Neuropathy	16 (39%)	12 (24.3%)	**<0.05**	**3.7 (1.3-10.38)**	**2.12 (1.19-3.76)**
Nephropathy	24 (85.3%)	32 (95.4%)	NS	2.75(0.69-10.95)	1.19 (0.95-1.48)
PeripheralVascular Disease	15 (53.5%)	29 (78.3%)	NS	0.60 (0.22-1.62)	0.82 (0.55-1.22)
Osteomyelitis	12(35.7%)	31 (78.3%)	**<0.05**	**0.30 (0.11-0.85)**	**0.61 (0.38-0.977)**

n, number of patients; **BMI**, body mass index; **HbA1c**, glycated hemoglobin; **Se TC**, serum total cholesterol; **Se TAG**, serum triglycerides; **Se HDL-C**, high-density-lipoprotein-cholesterol; **Se LDL-C**, low-density lipoprotein-cholesterol; **OR**; odd ratio; **RR**, risk ratio; **CI**, confidence interval; **NS**, not significant.

4.4. Microbiological profile of Aerobic Bacteria by Conventional Microbiology:

Among the 90 DFU subjects studied, 70 ulcer specimens were processed for aerobic bacterial analysis. No growth was observed in 20 (22.2%) patients since the wounds were of grade 0 and non-infected, and 70 (77.7%) samples showed positive growth. Mono-microbial growth in 53 (75.7%) and 17 (24.2%) patients had poly-microbial infection.

Aerobic Bacterial Infection	N (%)
➢ Mono-microbial growth	53 (75.7%)
➢ Poly-microbial growth	17 (24.2%)

4.5. Profile of Aerobic Bacteria Isolated from DFUs:

A total of 87 aerobic isolates were identified from 70 ulcer specimens, averaging 1.2 species per lesion. Fifty-three (75.7%) had mono-microbial infection, and poly-microbial etiology was observed in 17 (24.3%) cases. In the present study Gram-negative bacilli were predominant (75.9%) than Gram-positive cocci (24.1%). In terms of relative abundance, *Escherichia coli* accounted for (19.5%), followed by *Staphylococcus aureus* (18.4%), *Pseudomonas aeruginosa* (17.2%), *Klebsiella species* (14.9%), *Citrobacter species* (12.6%), *Proteus species* (11.5%) and *Enterococcus faecalis* (5.7%). Table 20 shows the distribution of isolates obtained from 70 pus samples. Figure 11 & 12 shows growth of aerobic bacteria isolated from DFUs pus samples.

Table 19: Aerobic bacteria (N = 87) isolated from DFU pus samples

Name of isolates	N (%)
Escherichia coli	17 (19.5%)
Staphylococcus aureus	16 (18.4%)
Pseudomonas aeruginosa	15 (17.2%)
Klebsiella species	13 (14.9%)
Citrobacter species	11 (12.6%)
Proteus species	10 (11.5%)
Enterococcus faecalis	5 (5.7%)

N, number of isolates

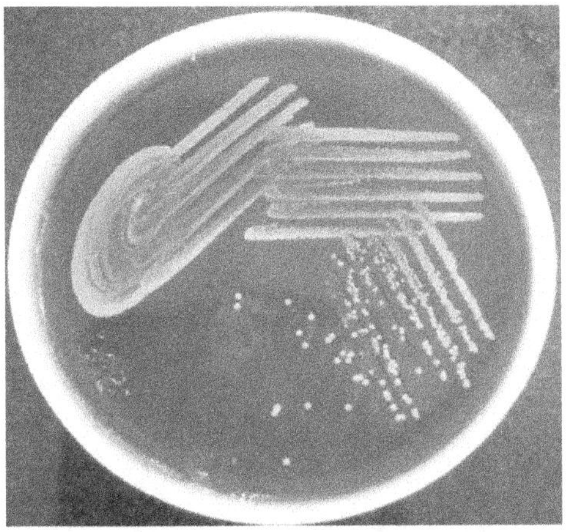

a) ***Staphylococcus aureus***

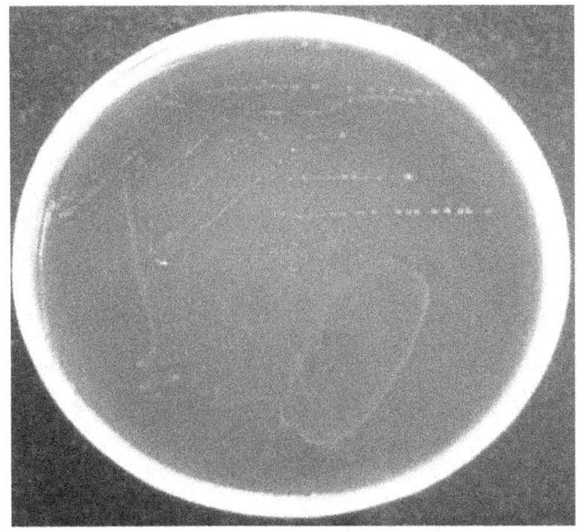

b) Enterococcus faecalis

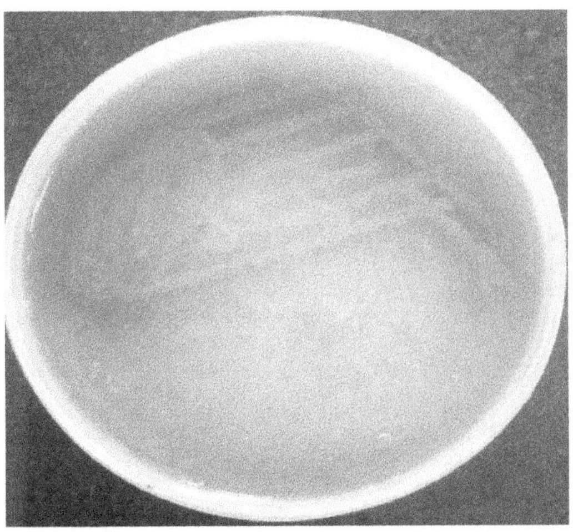

c) Pseudomonas aeruginosa

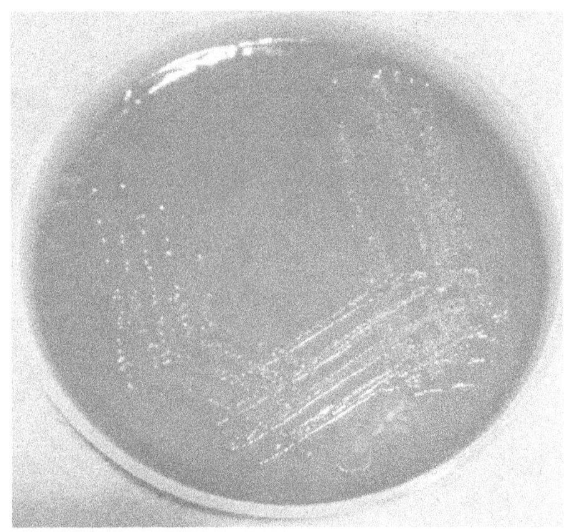

d) Citrobacter species

Figure 11: Growth of a) *Staphylococcus aureus* b) *Enterococcus faecalis* c) *Pseudomonas aeruginosa* d) *Citrobacter species.*

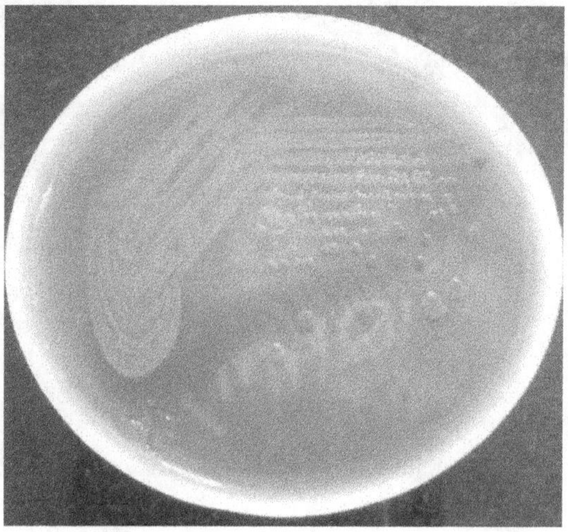

a) Escherichia coli

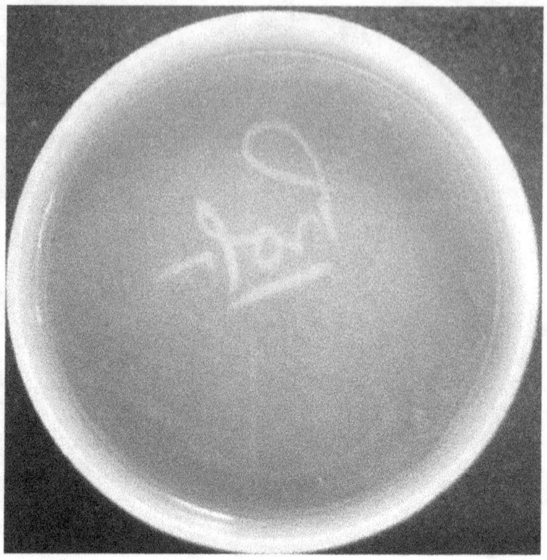

b) Proteus species

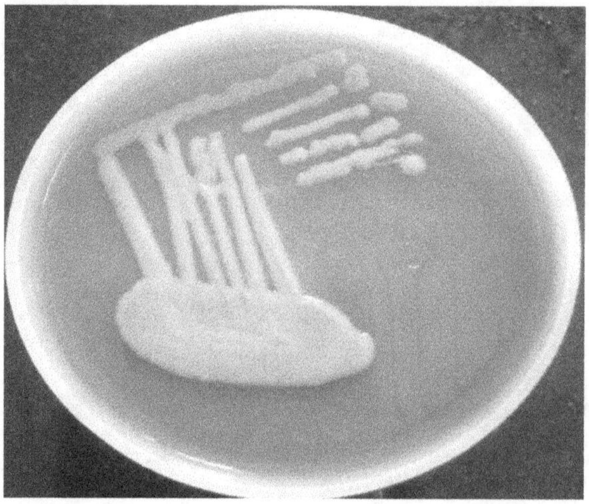

c) Klebsiella species

Figure 12: Growth of a) *Escherichia coli* b) *Proteus species* c) *Klebsiella species*

4.6. Profile of Aerobic Bacteria Isolated from different growth type:

In Gram-positive group, *Enterococcus faecalis* was found only in poly-microbial growth type. More than half of gram-negative aerobes showed mono-microbial growth pattern (60.9%). Among Gram-negative aerobes the most common isolates of mono-microbial infection were *Escherichia coli* (24.5%) followed by *Pseudomonas aeruginosa* (22.6%). In poly-microbial growth, the most commonly isolated gram-negative aerobes were *Citrobacter species*, *Proteus species,* 20.5% each followed by *Enterococcus faecalis* and *Klebsiella species*, 14.7% each (Table 21).

Table 20: Distribution of isolates in different growth types

S.No.	Name of isolates	Growth type	
		Mono-microbial	Poly-microbial
		N%	N%
1.	*Staphylococcus aureus*	12 (22.6%)	4 (11.7%)
2.	*Enterococcus faecalis*	0 (0%)	5 (14.7%)
3.	*Escherichia coli*	13 (24.5%)	4 (11.7%)
4.	*Pseudomonas aeruginosa*	12 (22.6%)	3 (8.8%)
5.	*Klebsiella species*	8 (15.1%)	5 (14.7%)
6.	*Citrobacter species*	4 (7.5%)	7 (20.5%)
7.	*Proteus species*	4 (7.5%)	7 (20.5%)
	Total	**53 (60.9%)**	**34 (39%)**

N, number of isolates

4.7. Distribution of Aerobic Bacterial Isolates among Wagner's grades:

The distribution of bacterial isolates among the different grades of DFU is listed in Table 22. Majority of bacteria were isolated from Grade III, 32 (36.7%); followed by 26 (29.8%) in Grade IV, 16 (18.3%) in Grade II, 13 (14.9%) in Grade I. The most common isolates of grade I was *Staphylococcus aureus* (30.7%) followed by *Citrobacter species* (23%). In grade II, *Staphylococcus aureus* and *Escherichia coli* were predominantly present (25% each). *Escherichia coli* (21.8%) and *Pseudomonas aeruginosa* (18.7%) were common isolates of grade III ulcers followed by *Staphylococcus aureus* and *Proteus species,* (15.6% each). In grade IV ulcers the most commonly isolated bacteria were *Klebsiella species* and *Proteus species*, (19.2% each).

Table 21: Distribution of isolates in different Wagner's Grade

S.No.	Name of isolates	Grade I	Grade II	Grade III	Grade IV	Total
		N (%)	N (%)	N (%)	N (%)	N (%)
1.	*Staphylococcus aureus*	4 (30.7%)	4 (25%)	5 (15.6%)	3 (11.5%)	16 (18.3%)
2.	*Enterococcus faecalis*	0 (0%)	1 (6.2%)	2 (6.2%)	2 (7.6%)	5 (5.7%)
3.	*Escherichia coli*	2 (15.3%)	4 (25%)	7 (21.8%)	4 (15.3%)	17 (19.5%)
4.	*Pseudomonas aeruginosa*	2 (15.3%)	3 (18.7%)	6 (18.7%)	4 (15.3%)	15 (17.2%)
5.	*Klebsiella species*	2 (15.3%)	2 (12.5%)	4 (12.5%)	5 (19.2%)	13 (14.9%)
6.	*Citrobacter species*	3 (23.0%)	2 (12.5%)	3 (9.3%)	3 (11.5%)	11 (12.6%)
7.	*Proteus species*	0 (0%)	0 (0%)	5 (15.6%)	5 (19.2%)	10 (11.4%)
	Total	**13(14.9%)**	**16(18.3%)**	**32(36.7%)**	**6(29.8%)**	**87**

N, number of isolates

4.8. Frequency of Distribution of Bacteria among Healing and Non-Healing Ulcer Group:

A total of 50 (57.4%) isolates were identified from patients with non-healing ulcers and 37 (42.5%) from those with healing wounds. Among the gram-positive bacteria, 66.6% were isolated from non-healing ulcers and 33.3% from healing lesions, whereas 54.5% of gram-negative bacteria were identified from non-healing ulcers, and 45.5% from healing ones. A detailed picture of all the bacteria from both groups is depicted in Table 23. Subjects with non-healing ulcers during hospital stay had a predominance of *Escherichia coli* and *Pseudomonas aeruginosa* (13.8% each), followed by *Staphylococcus aureus* (12.6%). *Klebsiella species* (10.3%), followed by *Citrobacter species* (9.2%) were most frequent in healing wounds. Those with healing ulcers had predominance of *Klebsiella species* (10.6%) followed by *Citrobacter species* (9.1%), *Staphylococcus aureus*, *Escherichia coli* and *Proteus species* (5.7% each).

Table 22: Distribution of Isolates in Subjects with Healing and Non-Healing Ulcers

S.No.	Name of isolates	Total (n= 70) N (%)	Healing ulcers (n= 27) N (%)	Non-Healing ulcers (n= 43) N (%)
1.	*Staphylococcus aureus*	16 (18.3%)	5 (5.7%)	11 (12.6%)
2.	*Enterococcus faecalis*	5 (5.7%)	2 (2.3%)	3 (3.4%)
3.	*Escherichia coli*	17 (19.5%)	5 (5.7%)	12 (13.7%)
4.	*Pseudomonas aeruginosa*	15 (17.2%)	3 (3.4%)	12 (13.7%)
5.	*Klebsiella species*	13 (14.9%)	9 (10.3%)	4 (4.5%)
6.	*Citrobacter species*	11 (12.6%	8 (9.1%)	3 (3.4%)
7.	*Proteus vulgaris*	10 (11.4%)	5 (5.7%)	5 (5.7%)

n, number of subjects; **N**, number of isolates

4.9. Antimicrobial Susceptibility profile of Aerobic Isolates:

4.9.1. Antibiogram of Gram-positive-cocci:

As regards to the antibiotic resistance pattern of gram-positive cocci, more than 65% strains of *Staphylococcus aureus* were resistant to levofloxacin (56.1%) followed by gentamicin (39.1%) and erythromycin (39.1%). All the isolates of gram-positive cocci were sensitive towards vancomycin (100%), amikacin (90.5%) and ciprofloxacin (71.4%). MRSA accounted for 25% of isolated strains of *Staphylococcus aureus* and were resistant to oxacillin (Table 24).

Table 23: Antibiogram of Gram-positive cocci

Antibiotics	*Staphylococcus aureus* (N = 16)		*Enterococcus faecialis* (N = 5)		Total (N = 21)	
	S (%)	R (%)	S (%)	R (%)	S (%)	R (%)
Amikacin	14 (87.5%)	2 (12.5%)	5 (100%)	0 (0%)	19 (90.5%)	2 (9.5%)
Erythromycin	10 (62.5%)	6 (37.5%)	4 (80%)	1 (20%)	14 (66.7%)	7 (33.3%)
Ciprofloxacin	11 (68.75%)	5 (31.25%)	4 (80%)	1 (20%)	15 (71.4%)	6 (28.6%)
Gentamicin	10 (62.5%)	6 (37.5%)	4 (80%)	1 (20%)	14 (66.7%)	7 (33.3%)
Levofloxacin	6 (37.5%)	10 (62.5%)	4 (80%)	1 (20%)	10 (47.6%)	11(52.4%)
Oxacillin	11 (68.75%)	5 (31.25%)	5 (100%)	0 (0%)	16 (76.2%)	5 (23.8%)
Vancomycin	16 (100%)	0 (0%)	5 (100%)	0 (0%)	21 (100%)	0 (0%)

N, number of isolates; **S,** sensitive; **R,** resistant

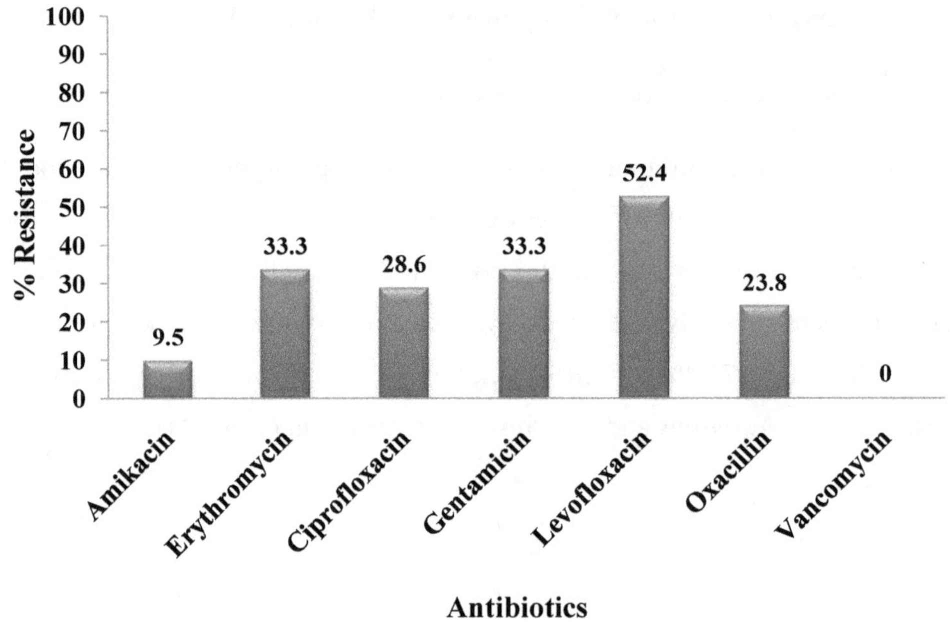

Figure 13: Antibiogram of Gram-positive cocci

4.9.2. Antibiogram of *Enterobacteriaceae:*

In *Escherichia coli*, the majority of strains were resistant to cefoperazone (82.3%), followed by gentamicin, levofloxacin, and tobramycin (70.6% each). *Klebsiella species* were found to be highly resistant to cefixime (84.6%) and cefoperazone (69.2%). *Citrobacter species* showed highest resistance to cefoperazone (81.8%) and ceftriaxone (81.8%), while resistance to gentamicin and cefepime was 63.6% each. High level of resistance to amikacin, cefoperazone, and tobramycin (70% each) was found in *Proteus species* (Table 25).

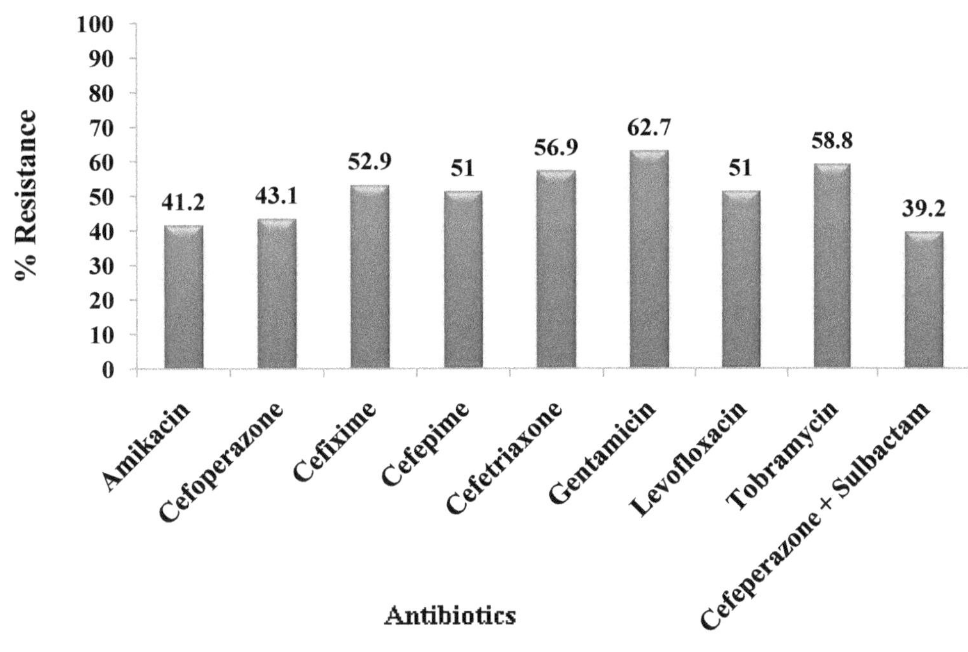

Figure 14: Antibiogram of *Enterobacteriaceae*

Table 24: Antibiogram of *Enterobacteriaceae*

Antibiotics	***Escherichia coli*** **(N = 17)**		***Klebsiella species*** **(N = 13)**		***Citrobacter species*** **(N = 11)**		***Proteus species*** **(N = 10)**		**Total (N = 51)**	
	S (%)	R (%)	S (%)	R (%)	S (%)	R (%)	S (%)	R (%)	S (%)	R (%)
Amikacin	13(76.5%)	4(23.5%)	9(69.2%)	4(30.8%)	5 (45.4%)	6(54.5%)	3 (30%)	7(70%)	30(58.8%)	21(41.2%)
Cefoperazone	3(17.6%)	14(82.3%)	4(30.8%)	9 (69.2%)	2(18.2%)	9(81.8%)	3 (30%)	7(70%)	15(29.4%)	22(43.1%)
Cefixime	6(35.3%)	11(64.7%)	2 (15.4%)	11(84.6%)	10(90.9%)	1 (9.0%)	6 (60%)	4(40%)	24(47.0%)	27(52.9%)
Cefepime	6(35.3%)	11(64.7%)	10(76.9%)	3(23.1%)	4 (36.4%)	7(63.6%)	5 (50%)	5(50%)	25(49.0%)	26(51.0%)
Cefetriaxone	6 (35.3%)	11(64.7%)	10(76.9%)	3(23.1%)	2 (18.2%)	9(81.8%)	4 (40%)	6(60%)	22(43.1%)	29(56.9%)
Gentamicin	5 (29.4%)	12(70.6%)	6(46.15%)	7(53.8%)	4 (36.4%)	7(63.6%)	4 (40%)	6(60%)	19(37.2%)	32(62.7%)
Levofloxacin	5(29.4%)	12(70.6%)	10(76.9%)	3(23.1%)	6 (54.5%)	5(45.4%)	4 (40%)	6(60%)	25(49.0%)	26(51.0%)
Tobramycin	5(29.4%)	12(70.6%)	6(46.15%)	7(53.8%)	6 (54.5%)	5(45.4%)	3 (30%)	7(70%)	20(39.2%)	30(58.8%)
Cefeperazone + Sulbactam	8(47.0%)	9(52.9%)	12(92.3%)	1 (7.7%)	5 (45.4%)	6(54.5%)	6 (60%)	4(40%)	31(60.8%)	20(39.2%)

N,numberofisolates; **S**, sensitive; **R**, resistant

4.9.3. Antibiogram of *Pseudomonas aeruginosa*:

Among the isolates of *Pseudomonas aeruginosa*, piperacillin (53.3%) and piperacillin+tazobactam (86.6%) showed good activity. All strains of *Pseudomonas aeruginosa* were found to be sensitive to imipenem (Table 26).

Table 26: Antibiogram of *Pseudomonas aeruginosa*

Antibiotics	*Pseudomonas aeruginosa* (N = 15)	
	S (%)	**R (%)**
Amikacin	5 (33.3%)	10 (66.7%)
Ceftazidime	4 (26.7%)	11 (73.3%)
Cefepime	4 (26.7%)	11 (73.3%)
Levofloxacin	6 (40.0%)	9 (60.0%)
Sparfloxacin	4 (26.7%)	11 (73.3%)
Tobramycin	5 (33.3%)	10 (66.7%)
Piperacillin	8 (53.3%)	7 (46.7%)
Piperacillin+Tazobactam	12 (80.0%)	3 (20.0%)
Imipenem	15 (100%)	0 (0%)

N, number of isolates; **S**, sensitive; **R**, resistant

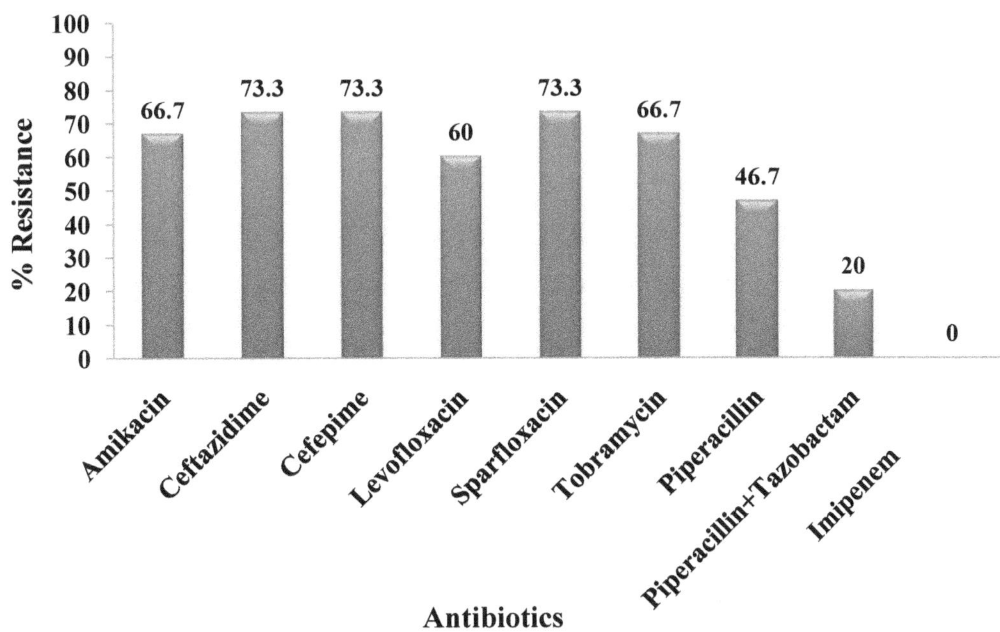

Figure 15: Antibiogram of *Pseudomonas aeruginosa*

4.10. Identification of pathogens by PCR:

The results of the present study reported the most commonly found aerobic bacteria infecting DFUs in northern India. Table 27 shows the distribution of common pathogens found in infected diabetic foot wounds of 70 patients.

Ninety patients suffering from DFUs were admitted to endocrinology ward. Seventy samples showed positive growth by conventional methodologies. All wound samples were identified positive by PCR and the most prevalent isolates identifiable by PCR were *Pseudomonas aeruginosa* (26.8%), *Escherichia coli* (25.6%), *Staphylococcus aureus* (24.3%), *and Klebsiella species* (23.1%).

Table 26: Frequency of organisms detected by PCR

Microorganisms	N	%
Staphylococcus aureus	20	24.3
Klebsiella species	19	23.1
Pseudomonas aeruginosa	22	26.8
Escherichia coli	21	25.6
Total	**82**	

N, number of isolates

Table 28 shows a comparison of frequency of isolates detected both from bacteriological methods and PCR. The most frequent bacteria detected both by PCR and bacteriological assay was *Escherichia coli* accounting 21 (26.8%) and 17 (27.8%) respectively. The frequency of *Staphylococcus aureus* according to culture, was 16 (26.2%) and 20 (24.3%) strains of it were detected by PCR. Similarly, there were 15 (23.5%) strains of *Pseudomonas aeruginosa* identifiable by culture whereas PCR detected 22 (26.8%) strains of this isolate. *Klebsiella species* was least frequent when analyzed both by culture based methods, 13 (21.3%) and PCR, 19 (23.1%).

Table 27: Comparison between the Frequencies of Isolates Detected by Conventional Methods and PCR

Microorganisms	Conventional N (%)	PCR N (%)
Staphylococcus aureus	16 (26.2%)	20 (24.3%)
Klebsiella species	13 (21.3%)	19 (23.1%)
Pseudomonas aeruginosa	15 (24.5%)	22 (26.8%)
Escherichia coli	17 (27.8%)	21 (25.6%)
Total	**61**	**82**

N, number of isolates

All culture based wound samples had organisms that were identifiable by the PCR assays. PCR identified all organisms recovered from culture methods. Overall PCR targeted hundred percent of common aerobic organisms detected by culture based assays Additionally PCR assay identified DNA from 21 isolates which were not reported by wound cultures.

Table 28: Additional isolates identified by PCR

Microorganisms	N (%)
Staphylococcus aureus	4 (19.0%)
Klebsiella species	6 (28.5%)
Pseudomonas aeruginosa	7 (33.3%)
Escherichia coli	4 (19.0%)
Total	**21**

N, number of isolates

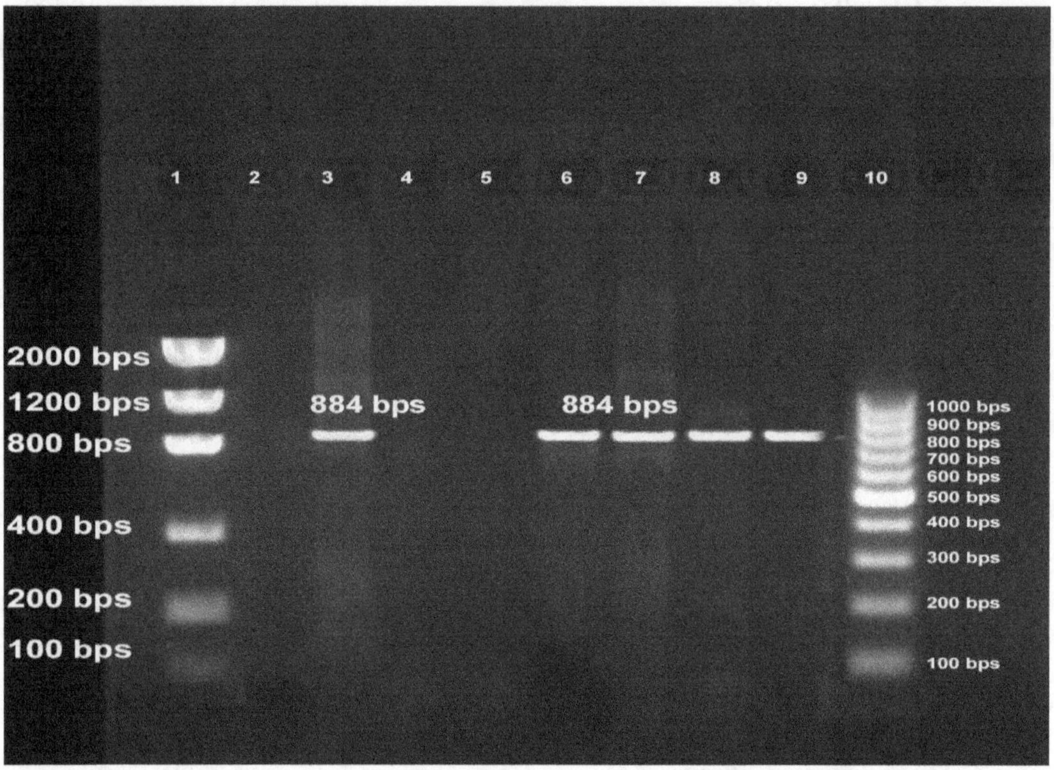

Figure 16: Gel image showing specific amplification of *Escherichia coli*. Amplified products of each reaction were analyzed by electrophoresis on Ethidium bromide stained 2% agarose gels. The band in each well corresponds to the PCR

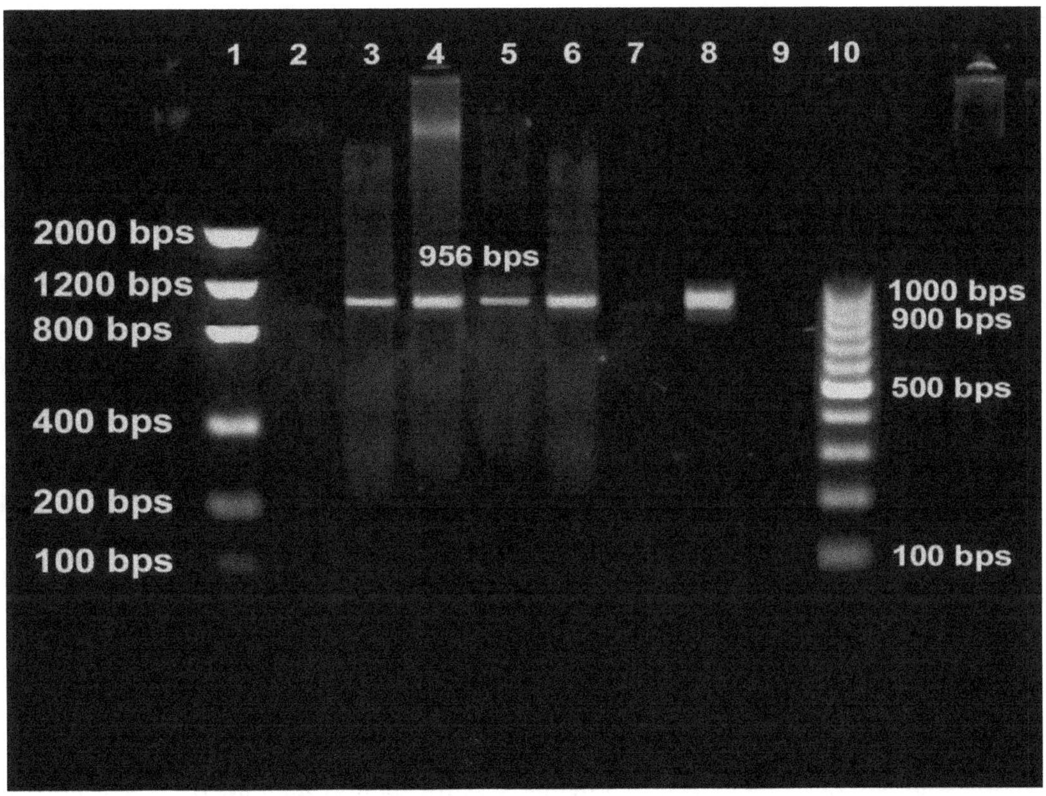

Figure 17: Gel image showing specific amplification of *Pseudomonas aeruginosa*. Amplified products of each reaction were analyzed by electrophoresis on Ethidium bromide stained 2% agarose gels. The band in each well corresponds to the PCR

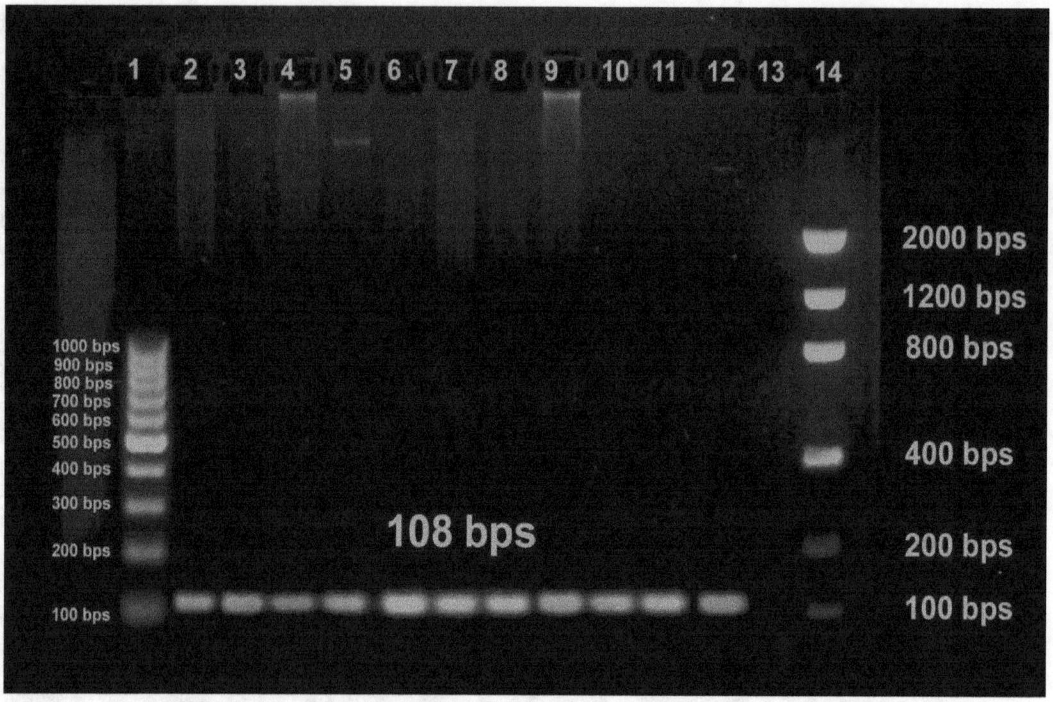

Figure 18: Gel image showing specific amplification of *Klebsiella species.* Amplified products of each reaction were analyzed by electrophoresis on Ethidium bromide stained 2% agarose gels. The band in each well corresponds to the PCR

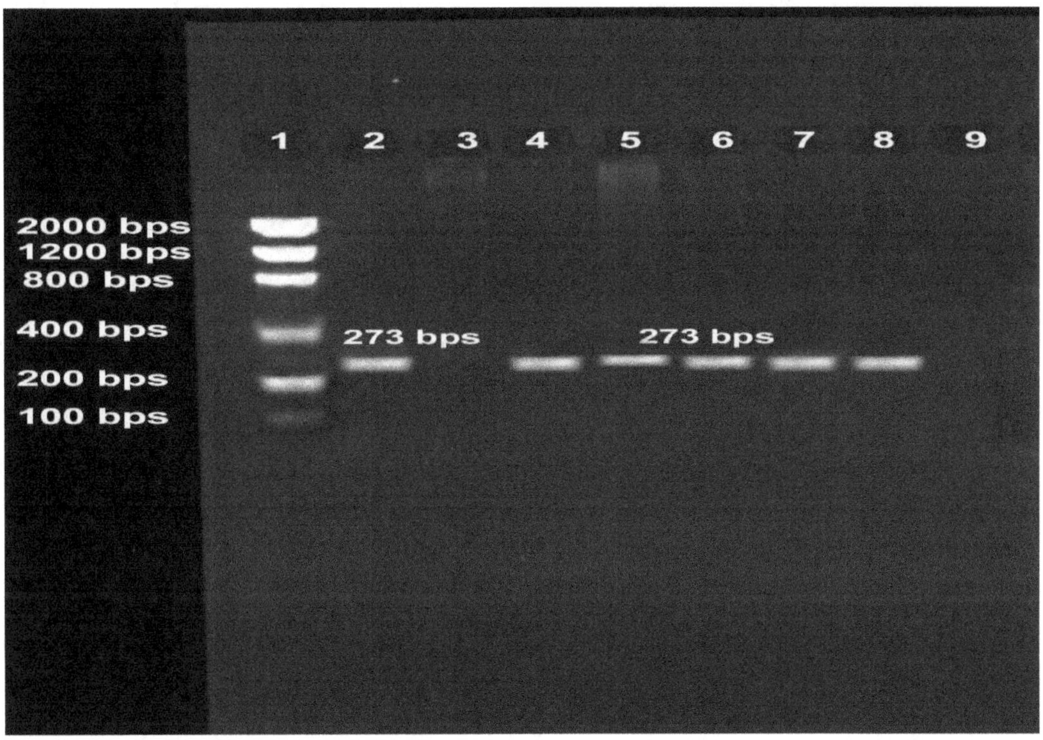

Figure 19: Gel image showing specific amplification of *Staphylococcus aureus*. Amplified products of each reaction were analyzed by electrophoresis on Ethidium bromide stained 2% agarose gels. The band in each well corresponds to the PCR

4.11. Inflammatory Markers in Diabetic Foot Subjects:

4.11.1. Immune Mediators in Control and Diabetic Foot Group:

Subjects with DFUs had significantly raised plasma immune mediators like neutrophils (49.9 ± 18.1 v/s 25.9 ± 16.5; $p < 0.05$), cytokines, IL-6 (69.5 ± 21.5 ng/mL v/s 29.7 ±10.8 ng/mL, $p < 0.05$), IL-8 (50.1 ng/mL ± 18.9 v/s 35.4 ± 8.9 ng/mL, $p < 0.05$), and TNF-α (56.6 ± 23.9 ng/mL v/s 37.5 ± 9.9 ng/mL, $p < 0.05$) than control subjects respectively. NF-κB (87.0 ± 29.1 ng/mL v/s 67.2 ± 11.3 ng/mL, $p < 0.05$) and pro-calcitonin (3.8 ± 2.1 pg/mL v/s 1.32 ± 0.98 pg/mL, $p < 0.05$) levels were also significantly higher in diabetic foot subjects than control group. However, no significant changes in level of lymphocyte percentage, IL-1-β and MCP-1 were observed in two groups (Table 30).

Table 29: Plasma Immune Mediators in Control and Diabetic Foot Group

Inflammatory markers	Control group (n= 40)	DFU group (n=70)	*p value*
Lymphocytes (%)	23.2 ± 8.1	25.9 ± 16.5	0.3347
Neutrophils (%)	25.9 ± 16.5	49.9 ± 18.1	0.0001
IL-6 (ng/mL)	29.7 ±10.8	69.5 ± 21.5	0.0001
IL-8 (ng/mL)	35.4 ± 8.9	50.1 ± 18.9	0.0001
IL- 1β (ng/mL)	31.0 ± 7.3	35.0 ± 14.3	0.102
TNF-α (ng/mL)	37.5 ± 9.9	56.6 ± 23.9	0.0001
NF-κB (ng/mL)	67.2 ± 11.3	87.0 ± 29.1	0.0001
MCP-1 (ng/mL)	88.7 ± 32.4	75.6 ± 35.6	0.107
Pro-calcitonin (pg/mL)	1.32 ± 0.98	3.8 ± 2.1	0.0001

n, number of subjects; **IL-6**, interleukin-6; **IL-8**, interleukin-8; **IL-1β**, interleukin-1 beta; **TNF-α**, tumor necrosis factor alpha; **NF-κB**, necrosis factor B; **MCP-1**, monocyte chemoattractant protein-1,

4.11.2. Immune Mediators in different Wagner's Grade (I-IV) of DFUs:

Diabetic patients with foot ulcers with increasing grade showed an up-regulation of circulating levels of cytokines, and chemokines. In the study, significantly increased levels of neutrophils (65.2 ± 20.5 v/s 38.1 ± 19.6, $p < 0.05$), TNF-α (68.2 ± 25.6 ng/mL v/s 35.5 ± 11.3 ng/mL, $p < 0.05$) and MCP-1 (99.1 ± 24.2 ng/mL v/s 67.2 ± 26.7 ng/mL, $p < 0.05$) between Grade III and Grade I respectively were found. In unadjusted analyses, patients with foot wounds of Wagner's Grade IV had significantly raised levels of lymphocytes (35.9 ± 10.4 ng/mL v/s 21.6 ± 12.7 ng/mL, $p < 0.05$), TNF-α (69.8 ± 28.7 ng/mL v/s 35.5 ± 11.3 ng/mL, $p < 0.05$), MCP-1 (99.4 ± 22.6 ng/mL v/s 67.2 ± 26.7 ng/mL) and pro-calcitonin (5.6 ± 2.3 pg/mL v/s 2.7 ± 1.8 pg/mL, $p < 0.05$) compared with patients of Grade I (Table 31).

Table 30: Plasma Immune Mediators in different Grades (I-IV) of DFUs

Inflammatory markers	Grade I (n= 3)	Grade II (n= 24)	Grade III (n= 19)	Grade IV (n=24)
Lymphocytes (%)	21.6 ± 12.7	27.5 ± 10.2	25.6 ± 9.3	35.9 ± 10.4•
Neutrophils (%)	38.1 ± 19.6	48.7 ± 18.1	65.2 ±20.5•	61 ± 20.3
IL-6 (ng/mL)	62.4 ± 28.4	70.5 ± 22.5	75.2 ± 27.5	69.9 ± 26.3
IL-8 (ng/mL)	50.5 ± 20.2	62.5 ± 32.5	55.8 ± 17.8	57.2 ± 18.7
IL- 1β (ng/mL)	31.4 ± 12.6	35.6 ± 22.3	38.7 ± 21.2	34.3 ± 15.6
TNF-α (ng/mL)	35.5 ± 11.3	55.4 ± 21.6	68.2 ± 25.6•	69.8 ± 28.7•
NF-κB (ng/mL)	71.3 ± 28.9	89.2 ± 23.8	88.8 ± 27.2	98.7 ± 30.8
MCP-1 (ng/mL)	67.2 ± 26.7	79.7 ± 30.2	99.1 ± 24.2	99.4 ± 22.6•
Pro-calcitonin (pg/mL)	2.7 ± 1.8	3.1 ±1.12	4.01 ± 2.2	5.6 ± 2.3•

n, number of subjects; **IL-6,** interleukin-6; IL-8, interleukin-8; **IL-1β**, interleukin-1 beta; **TNF-α**, tumor necrosis factor alpha; **NF-κB**, necrosis factor B; **MCP-1**, monocyte chemoattractant protein-1.

$p^{\bullet}$ when compared with Grade I

4.11.3. Immune Mediators in Subjects with Healing and Non-Healing Ulcers:

Patients with non-healing ulcers had significantly higher levels of IL-6 (88.9 ± 20.1 ng/mL v/s 50.1 ± 19.8 ng/mL, $p < 0.05$), IL-1β (28.7 ± 9.2 ng/mL v/s 41.3 ± 11.9 ng/mL, $p < 0.05$), TNF - α (63.3 ± 21.2 ng/mL v/s 49.9 ± 15.4 ng/mL NF-κB (80.1 ± 20.9 ng/mL v/s 70.4 ± 17.5 ng/mL, $p < 0.05$), MCP-1 (95.7 ± 29.3 ng/mL v/s 75.6 ± 33.2 ng/mL, $p < 0.05$) and pro-calcitonin (5.1 ± 1.57 pg/mL v/s 2.6 ± 1.2 pg/mL, $p < 0.05$) than healing ones respectively. No significant difference was observed in rest of the immune mediators.

Table 31: Plasma Immune Mediators in Subjects with Healing and Non-Healing Ulcers

Inflammatory markers	**Healing Ulcers** (n= 27)	**Non-healing Ulcers** (n= 43)	***p value***
Lymphocytes (%)	24.8 ± 10.8	27.0 ± 9.76	0.3814
Neutrophils (%)	54.2 ± 25.5	45.6 ± 21.6	0.1321
IL-6 (ng/mL)	50.1 ± 19.8	88.9 ± 20.1	0.0001
IL-8 (ng/mL)	55.6 ± 20.1	57.5 ± 22.3	0.7199
IL-1β (ng/mL)	28.7 ± 9.2	41.3 ± 11.9	0.0001
TNF-α (ng/mL)	49.9 ± 15.4	63.3 ± 21.2	0.0032
NF-κB (ng/mL)	70.4 ± 17.5	80.1 ± 20.9	0.0486
MCP-1 (ng/mL)	75.6 ± 33.2	95.7 ± 29.3	0.0009
Pro-calcitonin (pg/mL)	2.6 ± 1.2	5.1 ± 1.57	0.0001

n, number of subjects; **IL-6**, interleukin-6; **IL-8**, interleukin-8; **IL-1 β**, interleukin-1 beta; **TNF-α**, tumor necrosis factor alpha; **NF-κB**, necrosis factor B; **MCP-1**, monocyte chemoattractant protein-1.

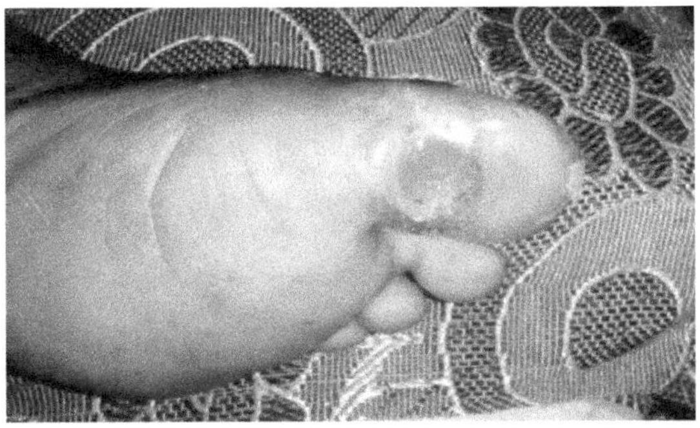

a) Image of Grade I ulcer

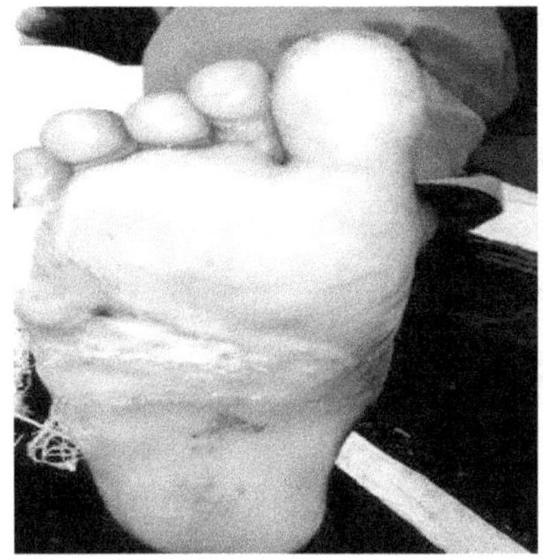

b) Image of Grade II ulcer

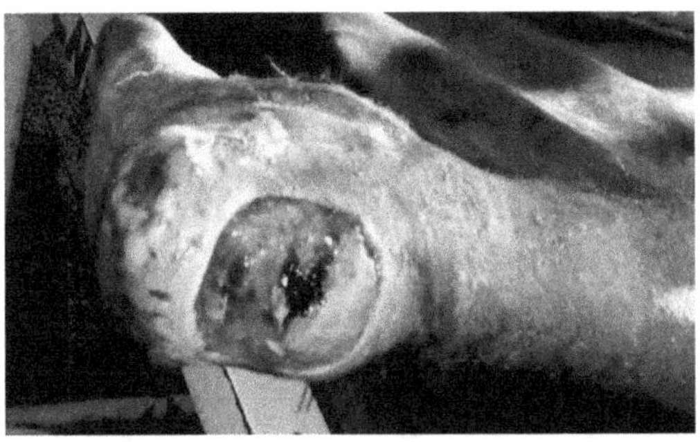

c) Image of Grade III ulcer

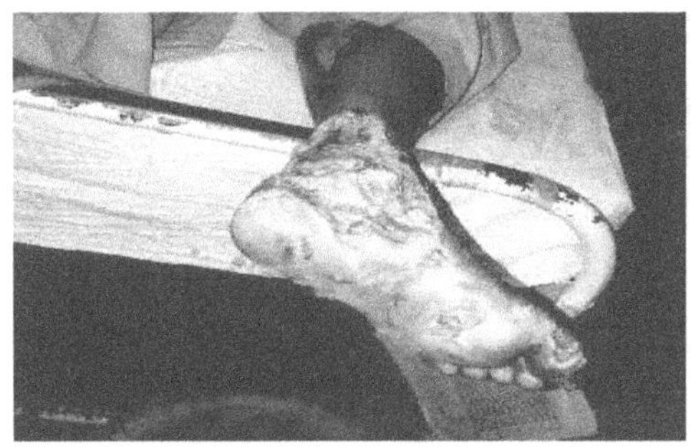

d) Image of Grade IV ulcer

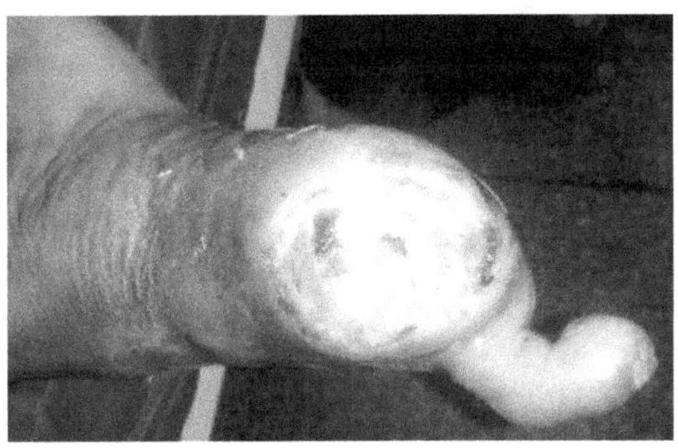

e) Amputated great toe

Figure 20: Images of Diabetic Foot Ulcers

Discussion

5. DISCUSSION

This study presents a comprehensive clinico-microbial profile of infections in DFUs hospitalized patients in a tertiary care hospital with special reference to identification of most prevalent isolates in infected DFUs by PCR.

With the rise in prevalence of DM globally, more so in developing countries, there is increasing problems of infections among patients especially those of lower limb ulcers which according to many studies accounts for 20% of total hospital admission and 85% of lower limb amputations (Adler et al., 1999). As pathogens of DFI plays a crucial role in changing the pathological-aspect of foot, efforts are made to study the profile of microbial flora harboring the wound and to study the associations of various clinical variables with non-healing state of ulcers.

In this prospective hospital based study, all diabetic subjects with infected foot ulcers were evaluated and various risk factors linked with this complication were assessed. Males were predominant which is in accordance with many earlier studies like of Abdulrazak et al., 2005; Gadepalli et al., 2005; Raja et al., 2007. It is possible to suggest that males are more liable to get foot ulcerations because of hindered joint mobility and higher foot pressure in addition to outdoor activities (Gadepalli et al., 2006; Kiziltan et al., 2007). Average age of subjects in this study was in range from 41-80 years in majority of cases, which is in accordance with studies reported by many authors (Apelqvist and Agardh 1992; Hokkam et al., 2009), which may be due to longer life span in this region. Majority of subjects enrolled had long standing diabetes $\geq$ 10 years which in consistent with Oyibo et al., 2001. In the present study majority of subjects had poor glycemic status (HbA1c) at the time of admission, and our findings were similar to reports of Gadepalli et al., 2006 and Zubair et al., 2010. This study showed a higher prevalence of osteomyelitis. The possible reason could be that most of the subjects are usually presented in tertiary care hospitals with Grade III and Grade IV. Lack of awareness and education regarding diabetic complications such as DFUs makes them susceptible to osteomyelitis. Patients with increased BMI (> 25 kg/m^2) were predominant, making obese patients having significantly higher risk for ulceration than normal-weight individuals. Our finding is in tune with earlier reports of Sohn et al., 2012, explaining a positive association of BMI with risk of developing foot ulcerations. DFU patients had a higher prevalence of neuropathy and vascular diseases making them key etiological agents involved in pathogenesis of DFU. Similarly other studies reported a higher prevalence of neuropathy and vasculopathy among DFU patients (Zubair et al., 2011).

Higher prevalence of PVD in our study is similar to previous studies (Prompers et al., 2008; Gadepalli et al., 2006), exposing PAD to be a limiting factor for healing. However, Parisi et al., 1980, reported no relationship between healing of a diabetic ulcer and peripheral vascular disease. This could be due to lower life expectancy of diabetics in developing countries compared to the Western areas.

Previous studiesfrom developing countries reported association between peripheral neuropathy and non-healing diabetic ulcers (Parisi et al., 1980; Musa et al., 2012). Few reports suggest that presence of neuropathy may directly affect the dernervation which contribute to impaired wound healing in diabetics (Richards et al., 1999; Gibran et al., 2002). In our study, the blend of peripheral neuropathy and ischemia was the commonest predictor of non-healing DFU. Loss of sensation and PAD were associated with a poorer outcome in these patients, suggesting that loss of protective sensation is not only a key factor in the development of an ulcer but also affects its outcome (Zubair et al., 2011). Inadequate blood supply due to atherosclerotic peripheral arteries leads to poor wound healing and lack of sensation causing repetitive traumas which are adversely treated with antimicrobials thereby leads to development of muti-drug resistant organisms (MDROs) in DFIs (Gadepalli et al., 2006). The ulcers with no classical signs of wound healing on routine monitoring were graded as non-healing types. The significant factors associated with development of non-healing lesions were older age, longer duration (>1 month) and increased ulcer size. In addition, altered lipid spectra (serum TAC > 150 mg/dL, serum TAG > 200 mg/dL, serum HDL-C < 40 mg/dL), higher prevalence of hypertension, neuropathy and peripheral vascular disease were linked to developing non-healing ulcers. Diabetes typically exhibits mixed dyslipidemia characterized by elevated TAGs and LDL-C and low levels of HDL-C. These lipid abnormalities and high serum cholesterol have proven to be major risk factor for cardio-vascular disease and have commonly being linked to worst outcomes (Nordergaard et al., 2007). In the present study the altered levels of triglycerides, cholesterol, LDL- C, HDL-C were associated with risk of developing non-healing diabetic lesions.

The local ulcer characteristics, that is, size and duration with location were found to have a significant effect on delayed wound healing. Our study found increasing ulcers size and depth involving bone along with duration of lesion were confounding factors associated with non-healing wounds. Similar findings were demonstrated by Parsi et al., 1980, reporting deferred healing in deeper ulcers of long duration. The deeper the ulcer is penetrating through the dermis, there is added tissue damage and necrosis favoring non-healing state (Lipsky et al., 2012). In our study majority of non-healing ulcers were present on heel of foot. Our finding were similar to Edmonds et al., 2006, stating the poor healing of ulcers on heel which are most likely to be ischemic. However, Bakheit et al., 2012, reported that heel ulcers are not associated with non-healing state. Ulcers on heel may be considered to have the poorest prognosis among DFU attributed by fat pad atrophy in people with diabetic neuropathy thereby reducing cushioning ability of heel (Edmonds et al., 2006).

Therefore, a typology of risk for non-healing ulcers in diabetic patients would be male patients with age more than 40 years, size of ulcer $\geq 4\ cm^2$, duration of ulcer > 1 month, heel ulcers and those with diabetic neuropathy, peripheral vascular disease and bone infection. These risk factors should be considered as indicating very high risk zone for diabetic patients and, in turn, signaling the need for close monitoring by health care professionals focusing non-healing ulcers.

DFIs are generally poly-microbial in nature (Sharma et al., 2006), but in our study mono-microbial etiology were found in 53% of cases, with the rate of isolation 1.24 bacteria per-patient which is lower than the previous studies (Gadepalli et al., 2006) which showed the rate of isolation between 2.3-5.9%. The major infective organisms in DFUs in our series of patients appear to be different. We found gram-negative aerobic isolates as most frequent organisms which is in accordance with previous reports (Ramakant et al., 2011; Gadepalli et al., 2006). However, studies from Western countries show that gram-positive aerobes are pre-dominant organisms isolated from DFU (Dang et al., 2003; Citron et al., 2007; Lipsky et al., 1990; Grayson et al., 1995; Joseph Axler., 1990). The prevalence of gram-negative bacilli in this series of DFU unlike Western countries may be because of chronicity of ulcers due to prior use of antibiotic therapy where gram-negative bacilli especially members of *Enterobacteriaceae* pre-dominates. The environmental factors such as sanitary habits, e.g. use of water for peri-anal wash (ablution) after defecation leading to contamination of hands with fecal flora, may also be responsible for the increase in the prevalence of gram-negative organisms in developing world as compared with Western countries (Ramakant et al., 2011). In this study, the ratio of gram-negative to gram-positive aerobes was found to be 3.0, which are larger than reported by Gadepalli et al., 2006.

In non-healing ulcers, gram-negative isolates were most prevalent. The commonest of them was *Escherichia coli* and *Pseudomonas aeruginosa*. Gram-negative isolates are emerging dominants of infection in DFI according to studies (Gadepalli et al 2006). In countries with warm climates, gram-negative isolates (especially *Pseudomonas aeruginosa*) are more prevalent leading to chronic non-healing ulcers (Lipsky et al., 2012). Highly resistant strains of *Escherichia coli* (Extended spectrum β lactamases) and *Pseudomonas aeruginosa* to commonly used antibiotics could be a possible reason in treatment failure adding to chronicity of wounds.

There is a strong association between heavy anti-microbial consumption within population and the frequency of recovery of resistant bacteria (Enne et al., 2001). Cars et al., 2001, compared the non-hospital use of antibiotics in the 15 member states of European Union in 1997 and found that in 11 countries, the most commonly used antibiotic was broad-spectrum penicillin. Data on antibiotic sales is not publicly available in many countries, including India. The overall resistance in our patients was high. The gram-negative isolates showed high rates of anti-microbial resistance. The reason may be indiscriminate use of antibiotics in the community (Ramakant et al., 2011). Another possible reason could be that most of our patients presenting our centre from the referring hospitals using a combination of drugs of different anti-microbials empirically. And also the variation in infection control policies, different climatic conditions, and other unrecognized factors (Hart and Kariuki et al., 1997) play a significant role. The frequent and unnecessary uses of antibiotics result in selection favoring resistant bacteria. In this study history and discharge records showed overwhelming majority of DFU patients who referred to our centre had received an antibiotic treatment before. However, in rest of the cases, the antibiotic treatment history could not be retrieved because most of the patients were illiterate, and did not know much which antibiotic was prescribed and in what doses. Resistance to antibiotics is seen when they are used for prolonged period of time. This resistance is an acquired form rather than intrinsic one. The former develops following a mutation in the DNA of a micro-organism or by acquisition of a new DNA. Acquisition of new DNA is accomplished by genetic elements such as plasmids or transposons. Resistance plasmids may be approximately 10 resistance genes for various antibiotics. Bacteria can transmit these characteristics to other bacteria (Gold and Mollering, 1996). Infections in these foot ulcers are requiring a longer duration of treatment and the use of appropriate antibiotic in an appropriate dosage (Ray-makers et al., 2001). Insufficient blood flow which causes further hindered penetration of antibiotics into the wound and therefore, a delay in healing occurs (Parkhouse and LeQuesne., 1988).

Exploring the spectrum of microbes invading diabetic wounds is central need involving proper swab specimens obtained from wound after debridement. Infection is routinely confirmed by standard conventional bacteriological tools. From past many decades culture obtained from wound specimen is the only way to determine the causative pathogen (s) in a DFI. Tools of molecular genetics are advancing and microbial diversity of wounds can be more easily and sensitively explored by using molecular techniques than culture methodologies. Previous studies have compared phenotypic culturing to molecular methods (Rhoads et al., 2012). These studies reported that molecular microbial tests are more sensitive than culture testing and assures the improvement in patient care and therefore this study was performed to compare culturing to the molecular testing method, PCR. PCR is known to be more sensitive than culture for bacterial identification in clinical samples (Jalava et al., 2000 and Gurtner et al., 2001). The current study adds to this body of work. In our study we validated the protocols for identification of most common isolates of DFI using PCR and also reported the comparative evaluation of biochemical and PCR assays in exploring the commonest bacteria of DFUs.

As a proof of principle, we designed a panel of PCR assays to target the most clinically relevant aerobic bacterial pathogens commonly isolated from diabetic foot wounds based on culture based results from our patient population and previous published studies (Zubair et al., 2011; Gadepalli et al., 2006). The sensitivity of our PCR assays was tremendous compared to that of cultures. Under optimal conditions, the turnaround time for PCR results is between 4-6 hrs. Out of 70 DFU subjects, positive growth was observed in all samples by both bacteriological methods and PCR. Like previous studies, this study also demonstrates that culture based bacteriological testing and molecular testing of wound bacteria produces differing and often conflicting results because molecular methods are more sensitive than culture methods. It has been suggested that PCR fails to reach its speculative sensitivity because of the use of a small sample volume after a sequence of enzymatic cell lysis, which may or may not efficiently isolate the microbial DNA. The PCR assays identified DNA from 21 organisms that were not revealed by bacteriological method. There are several possible explanations for the culture-negative, PCR positive results, including: (i) a lack of sensitivity of cultures in poly-microbial settings, which has been previously reported in the setting of chronic wounds; or delay in processing of samples (Melendez et al., 2010). The other possible reason may be due to the fact that the bacteria were isolated from samples containing large number of other bacteria and they might not have been detected during initial screening due to competition of other numerous species and overgrowth on the selective/non-selective media by related micro-flora.

In this study, we showed that the PCR based bacterial identification system is useful for exploring of most clinically important bacterial strains with ambiguous biochemical profiles, and hence would be a useful substitution for conventional methodologies in identification of bacterial strains harboring DFUs. Additionally, this approach is hasty and uses instrumentation that is becoming more easily available in the clinical settings. Subsequent to the development of additional assays targeting clinically relevant aerobic organisms, we look forward to developing a rapid, cost-effective, clinically applicable molecular diagnostic panel to serve in the diagnosis and care of chronic wounds as risk of DFUs is increasing in developing countries.

It is very important to identify the causative pathogens from DFUs for many reasons. Majority of foot wounds in diabetics are non-healing, in which poor glycemic status, vascular disease, neuropathy along with repetitive ulcers plays major role. The halt in treatment with anti-microbial caused due to unavailability of culture report; worsen the wound status thereby making the situation unmanageable. Therefore in this study a primary protocol was established in our hospital for identifying the commonest bacteria prevalent in diabetic foot wounds according to previous published reports from northern India. In summary establishment in PCR based identification of common bacteria in clinical settings can be a valuable way due to short turnaround time and specific results.

Immune activation may precede the incidence of a DFU in the same way that it precedes the manifestation of type 2 diabetes and coronary heart disease. The status of the immune system may be relevant at several stages in development of chronic wounds. Given the surprising paucity of data on the role of systemic inflammation in DFUs, we evaluated the association between foot ulcers and immune status in diabetic patients with and without foot ulcers by measuring a range of immune mediators (cytokines and chemokines) representing different aspects of the immune system. Our study showed that diabetic patients with foot ulceration showed an up-regulation of circulating levels of cytokines, and chemokines and lower levels of certain immune mediators with diabetic patients without a history of foot ulcer. Severity of foot ulcer based on the Wagner's classification was associated with hiked levels immunological markers. Certain markers of inflammation were elevated in subjects with non-healing foot ulcers than those of healing status.

The finding of an altered immune status in patients with foot ulceration is interesting in several ways. First, only some markers of inflammation were up regulated (neutrophils, IL-6, IL-8, TNF-α, NF-κB and pro-calcitonin) in patients with DFU than control group, and others were not (lymphocytes, IL-1β and MCP-1). These results indicate a non-random and specific alteration of the immune state in DFU patients. Increase in the serum levels of cytokines have been associated with pathogenesis of diabetic associated complications (Muller et al., 2002) Chemokines aids the recruitment of leukocytes (such as neutrophils) to sites of injury and orchestrate the voyage of other cells like keratinocytes, endothelial cells, and fibroblasts during the different states of wound healing. Notably, this process is troubled in patients with diabetes, and a role of distorted chemokine expression in this context has been previously postulated (Muller et al., 2002). Although the presumed local expression of immune mediators does not necessarily translate into systemic concentrations, our results may reflect an amalgamation of normal and abnormal wound repair mechanisms. Firstly our study presents a comprehensive measurement of multiple immune mediators regulated independently from each other. Second, it aimed at determining the differences in levels of plasma immune mediators according to healing status. A novel observation of this study states that ulcers which failed the progressive healing had increased levels of TNF-α, MCP-1, IL-6 and NF-κB. In diabetes associated complications such as DFUs there is compromised delivery of nutrients to surrounding tissues, poor elimination of waste products and impaired wound healing along with immune alterations and increased susceptibility to infection (Vozarova et al., 2002). However, our data reveal that the elevated levels of inflammatory markers are mainly associated with the severity of ulceration and non-healing status. The characteristic of beneficial and deleterious immune mediators in the wound healing would be important to identify potential therapeutic targets and immuno-modulating treatment options. Our data also raises the possibility that inflammatory markers may provide an adjunctive method for early detection of this disease with non-healing wounds.

There are some **limitations** of this study. Information in neuropathic assessment, degree of blood pressure, lipid controls, previous record of hyperglycemia and antibiotic usage in all subjects in past was not available. To what extent these risk factors assessment has influenced the risk factors it is difficult to estimate. Other limitations of this study include the small size of the sample population, the lack of anaerobic bacteria cultures, and the difficulty of replicating this study at other laboratories. Only 70 subjects were examined in this study, which is not large sample size enough to recognize statistically significant trends, therefore multi-centric studies with large samples should be performed. The other shortcomings were, the panels of species selected for identification by PCR were less.

The potential limitations of immunological analysis are, the study is a prospective cohort study so that cause and effect, the association between systemic inflammation and foot ulcer cannot be investigated. This requires longitudinal studies to investigate the impact of inflammation on the development of foot lesions in diabetics and their prognostic values. Second, our study population reflected only patients with type 2 diabetes. The proportion of patients with type 1 diabetes was too small to run separate analyses. Therefore, our results are valid mainly for patients with type 2 diabetes as indicated by sensitivity analysis. Whether the observed results are specific for DFU or represent a common feature of impaired regeneration of chronic wounds cannot be inferred from our data as non-diabetic control group with chronic wounds was available, but the scarce data on systemic immune markers in non-diabetic chronic wounds indicate that at least some of the observed results may be characteristic of chronic ulcers in general. The two groups of patients studied were not matched for potential confounders such as age, duration, and type of diabetes, HbA1c, smoking habits, and cardiovascular risk factors. Furthermore, we cannot exclude confounding effects on immune reactions by psychic stress due to hospital admission and bed rest in patients with a foot ulcer, although bed rest seems to impair rather than activate immune function via modulation of cortisol levels.

References

Aalto AM, Uutela A, Aro AR. Health related quality of life among insulin-dependent diabetics: Disease-related and psychosocial correlates. *Patient Education and Counseling* 1997; 30:215–225

Abbas ZG, Archibald LK. Epidemiology of the diabetic foot in Africa. *Med Sci Monit* 2005; 11:262-270.

Abbott CA, Garrow AP, Carrington AL, et al. North-West Diabetes Foot Care Study. Foot ulcer risk is lower in South-Asian and African-Caribbean compared with European diabetic patients in the U.K.: the North-West Diabetes Foot Care Study. *Diabetes Care* 2005; 28:1869–1875.

Abdulrazak A, Bitar ZI, Al-Shamali AA, and Mobasher LA. Bacteriological study of diabetic foot infections. *J. Diabetes Complications* 2005; 19:138-141.

Abdulrazak A, Bitar ZI, Al-Shamali AA, et al. Bacteriological study of diabetic foot infections. *J Diabetes Complicat* 2005; 19:138–41.

Adler AI, Boyko EJ, Ahroni EH, et al. Lower-extremity amputation in diabetes: The independent effects of peripheral vascular disease, sensory neuropathy and foot ulcers. *Diabetes Care* 1999; 22:1029–35.

Adler AI, Boyko EJ, Ahroni J, et al. Lower extremity amputation in diabetes: the independent effects of peripheral vascular disease, sensory neuropathy, and foot ulcers. *Diabetes Care* 1999; 22:1029-1035.

Aguilar-Bryan L, Bryan J. Neonatal diabetes mellitus *Endocr. Rev* 2008; 29:265–291.

Ahuja MMS. Epidemiological studies on diabetes mellitus in India. In: Ahuja MMS, editor. Epidemiology of diabetes in developing countries. New Delhi: *Interprint* 1979; 29-38.

Aiello LP, Gardner TW, King GL, et al., Diabetic retinopathy. *Diabetes Care* 1998; 21:143–56.

Alsaad KO, Herzenberg AM. Distinguishing diabetic nephropathy from other causes of glomerulosclerosis: an update. *J Clin Pathol* 2007; 60:18–26.

American Diabetes Association. Implications of the Diabetes Control and Complications Trial. *Diabetes Care* 2000; 23:S24-S26.

American Diabetes Association. Standards of medical care in diabetes: 2007. *Diabetes Care* 2007;30:(suppl 1) S4-S41.

American Diabetes Association. Gestational diabetes mellitus. *Diabetes Care* 2003; 26(Suppl. 1):S103–S105.

American Diabetes Association: Consensus development conference on diabetic wound care. *Diabetes Care* 1999; 22:1354–1360.

Anandi C, Alaguraja D, Natarajan V, Ramanathan M, Subramaniam CS, Thulasiram M, et al. Bacteriology of diabetic foot lesions. *Indian J Med Microbiol* 2004; 22:175–8.

Apelqvist J, Agardh CD. The association between clinical risk factors and outcome of diabetic foot ulcers. *Diabetes Res Clin Pract* 1992; 18:43–53.

Apleqvist J, Larsson J, Agardh CD. Long term prognosis for patients with foot ulcers. *J. Intern. Med* 1993; 233:485-491.

Armstrong DG, Larvey LA, Harkless LB. Validation of wound classification system: the contribution of depth, infection, and ischemia to risk of amputation. *Diabetes Care* 1998; 21:855-859.

Armstrong DG, Larvey LA, Harkless LB. Validation of wound classification system: the contribution of depth, infection, and ischemia to risk of amputation. *Diabetes Care* 1998; 21:855-859.

Armstrong DG, Lavery LA. Diabetic foot ulcers: prevention, diagnosis and classification. *Am Fam Physician* 1998; 57:1325–32.

Armstrong DG, Lipsky BA. Advances in the treatment of diabetic foot infections. *Diabetes Technol Ther* 2004; 62:167-77.

Armstrong DG, Liswood PJ, Todd WF. Prevalence of mixed infections in the diabetic pedal wound: a retrospective review of 112 infections. 1995 William J. Stickel bronze award. *J Am Podiatr Med Assoc* 1995; 85:533–7.

Ashcroft FM. ATP-sensitive potassium channelopathies: focus on insulin secretion. *J. Clin. Invest* 2005; 115, 2047–2058.

Atkinson MA. The pathogenesis and natural history of type 1 diabetes. Cold Spring Harbor perspectives in medicine 2012; 2: a007641.

Bakheit HE, Mohamed MF, Mahadi SE et al. Diabetic heel ulcer in the Sudan: determinants of outcome. *J Foot Ankle Surg* 2012; 51:152–5.

Banerji MA, Chaiken RL, Huey H. GAD antibody negative NIDDM in adult black subjects with diabetic ketoacidosis and increased frequency of human leukocyte antigen DR3 and DR4. Flatbush diabetes. *Diabetes* 1994; 43:741–745.

Barrientos, S.; Stojadinovic, O.; Golinko, M.S.; Brem, H.; Tomic-Canic, M. Growth factors and cytokines in wound healing. *Wound Rep. Reg* 2008; 16:585–601.

Beach KW, Bedford GR, Bergelin RO, et al. Progression of lower-extremity arterial occlusive disease in type 2 diabetes mellitus. *Diabetes Care* 1998; 11:464–472.

Beckman JA, Ganz J, Creager MA, et al. Relationship of clinical presentation and calcification of culprit coronary artery stenoses. *Arterioscler Thromb Vasc Biol* 2001; 21:1618–22.

Beidler SK, Douillet CD, Berndt DF,. Inflammatory cytokine levels in chronic venous insufficiency ulcer tissue before and after compression therapy. *J Vasc Surg* 2009; 49:1013–20.

Bengtsson L, Jonsson M, Apelqvist J. Wound related pain is underestimated in patients with diabetic foot ulcers. *J Wound Care* 2008; 17:433–5.

Bogardus C, Lillioja S, Mott DM et al. Relationship between degree of obesity and in vivo insulin action in man. *Am. J. Physiol* 1985; 248:286-291.

Bottazzo GF, Florin-Christensen A, Doniach D. Islet-cell antibodies in diabetes mellitus with autoimmune polyendocrine deficiencies. *Lancet* 1974; 2:1279–1282.

Bottazzo GF, et al. In situ characterization of autoimmune phenomena and expression of HLA molecules in the pancreas in diabetic insulitis. *N Engl J Med* 1985; 313:353–360.

Boulton AJ, Vileikytel L, Ragnarson-Tennval G, et al. The global burden of diabetic foot disease. *Lancet* 2005; 366:1719–24.

Boulton AJM, Vileikyte L, Ragnarson – Tennvall G et al. The Global burden of diabetic foot disease. *Lancet* 2005; 366:1719-24.

Boulton AJM. The pathways to ulceration. The foot in Diabetes, 3rd ed.,pp. 19-31 edited by AJM Boulton, H Connor, and PR Cavangh, John Wiley and Sons, Chichseter, UK, 2000.

Bowler PG, Davies BJ. The microbiology of infected and noninfected leg ulcers. *International Journal of Dermatology* 1999; 38:573–578.

Boyko EJ, Ahroni JH, Smith DG, et al. Increased mortality associated with diabetic foot ulcer. *Diabetes Med* 1996; 13:967–72.

Boyko EJ, Ahroni JH, Stensel V, et al. A prospective study of risk factors for diabetic foot ulcer: the Seattle Diabetic Foot Study. *Diabetes Care* 1999; 22:1036- 42.

Boyko EJ, Ahroni JH, Stensel V, et al. A prospective study of risk factors for diabetic foot ulcer: the Seattle Diabetic Foot Study. *Diabetes Care* 1999; 22:1036-42.

Boyko EJ, Lipsky BA. Infection and diabetes mellitus. In Harris MI (ed): Diabetes in America, 2nd edition. NIH publication No 95-1468. Bethesda, MD: National Institute of Health. 1995:485-499.

Brodsky JW. The diabetic foot. In: Mann RA, Coughlin MJ, editors. Surgery of the foot and ankle. 7th ed., St Louis, MO: Mosby-Year Book; 1999.

Brownlee M, Aiello LP, Friedman E, Vinik AI, Nesto RW, Boulton AJM. Complications of Diabetes Mellitus. In: Williams Textboot of Endocrinology. 10th ed. 2003 (eds) Larsen R, Krokenberg HM, Melmed S, Polonsky KS. Suunders pp 1560-1563.

Brownlee M. Biochemistry and Molecular cell biology of diabetic complications. *Nature* 2001; 414:813-820.

Brownlee M. The patho-biology of diabetic complications: a unifying mechanism. *Diabetes* 2005; 54:1615–1625.

Buse JB, Rosenstock J. Prevention of cardiovascular outcomes in type 2 diabetes mellitus: trials on the horizon. *Endocrinol Metab Clin North Am* 2005; 34:221–35.

Cade WT Diabetes-related microvascular and macrovascular diseases in the physical therapy setting. *Phys Ther* 2008; 88:1322–1335.

Calhoun JH, Cantrell J, Cobos J, et al. Treatment of diabetic foot infections: Wagner classification, therapy, and outcome. *Foot Ankle* 1988; 9:101–6.

Campbell AJ, Busby WJ, Horwath CC et al. Relation of age, exercise, anthropometric measurements, and diet with glucose and insulin levels in a population aged 70 years and older. *American Journal Epidemiology* 1993; 138:688–696.

Caputo GM, Cavanagh PR, Ulbrecht JS, et al. Assessment and management of foot disease in patients with diabetes. *N Engl J Med* 1994; 331:854–860.

Carmeliet P. Angiogenesis in life, disease and medicine. *Nature* 2005; 438:932-936.

Carr DB, Gabbe S. Gestational diabetes: detection, management and implications. Clin *Diabetes* 1998; 16:4–11.

Cars O, Molstad S., Melander A. Variation in antibiotic use in the European Union. *Lancet* 2001; 357:1851–1883.

Centers for Disease Control and Prevention History of foot ulcer among persons with diabetes—United States, 2000–2002, MMWR *Morb Mortal Wkly Rep* 2003; 52:1098-102.

Chantelau E, Tanudjaja T, Altenhofer F, et al. Antibiotic treatment for uncomplicated neuropathic forefoot ulcers in diabetes: a controlled trial. *Diabet Med* 1996; 13:156–9.

Chen YQ, Su M, Walia RR et al. Sp1 sites mediate activation of the plasminogen activator inhibition-1 promoter by glucose in vascular smooth muscle cells. *J. Biol Chem* 1998; 273:8225-8231.

Chander Y, Ramakrishnan MA, Jindal N, Hansen K, Goyal SM. Differentiation of Klebsiella pneumoniae and K. oxytoca by multiplex polymerase chain reaction. Intern J *Appl Res Vet Med* 2011;9:138-142.

Coenye T, Goris J, Spilker T, Vandamme P, Li Puma JJ. Characterization of unusual bacteria isolated from respiratory secretions of cystic fibrosis patients and description of Inquilinus limosus gen. nov., sp. nov. *J. Clin. Microbiol* 2002;40:2062–2069.

Chen J, Griffiths MW. PCR differentiation of Escherichia coli from other gram-negative bacteria using primers derived from the nucleotide sequences flanking the gene encoding the universal stress protein. *Lett Appl Microbiol* 1998;27:369–71.

Cherry GC, Hughes MA, Ferguson MWJ, et al. Wound healing: In Morris PJ, Wood WC (eds): Oxford textbook of surgery. Oxford UK: Oxford University Press 2000:131-159.

Citron, DM, Goldstein EJ, Merriam CV et al., Bacteriology of moderate-to-severe diabetic foot infections and *In vitro* activity of antimicrobial agents. *J. Clin. Microbiol* 2007; 45:2819–2828.

Clark A, Wells CA, Buley ID, et al. Islet amyloid, increased A-cells, reduced B-cells and exocrine fibrosis: quantitative changes in the pancreas in type 2 diabetes. *Diabetes Res* 1988; 9:151–9.

Clinical and Laboratory Standards Institute. M2-A9. Performance standards for antimicrobial disk susceptibility tests; approved standard, 9th ed. Clinical and Laboratory Standards Institute, Wayne, PA. 2006.

CLSI. Abbreviated identification of Bacteria and Yeast; Approved guideline-Second edition. CLSI document M35-A2, Wayne PA: Clinical and Laboratory Standards Institute; 2008.

Coleman WC. Footwear considerations. In: The high-risk foot in diabetes mellitus. Frykberg RG (ed). Churchill Livingstone, New York 1990; 487-496.

Craven PA, Studer RK, DeRubertis FR. Impaired nitric oxide dependent cyclic guanosine monophosphate generation in glomeruli from diabetic rats. Evidence for Protein Kinase C –mediated suppression of the cholinergic response . *J. Clin. Invest* 1994; 93:311-320.

Cutting K, Harding K. Criteria for identifying wound infection. *J Wound Care* 1994; 3:198–201.

Dabelea D, Bell RA, et al. Incidence of diabetes in youth in the United States. *JAMA* 2007, 297:2716–2724.

Dang CN, Prasad YD, Boulton AJM, et al. Methicillin-resistant Staphylococcus aureus in the diabetic foot clinic: A worsening problem. *Diabet Med* 2003; 20:159-161.

Dang H & Lowell CR. Microbial surface colonization and biofilm development in marine environments. *Microbiol. Mol. Biol. Rev* 2016; 80:91–138.

Davey ME, O'Toole GA. Microbial biofilms: from ecology to molecular genetics. Microbiol. *Mol. Biol. Rev* 2000; 64:847–867.

Davies CE. The comprehensive analysis of the microbial community of clinically non-infected chronic venous leg ulcers. PhD thesis. Department of Oral Surgery, Medicine and Pathology, University of Wales College of Medicine, Cardiff, UK. 2003.

Davies CE. The comprehensive analysis of the microbial community of clinically non infected chronic venous leg ulcers. PhD thesis. Department of Oral Surgery, Medicine and Pathology, University of Wales College of Medicine, Cardiff, UK. 2003.

Day MR, Armstrong DG. Factors associated with methicillin resistance in diabeticfoot infections. *Journal of Foot and Ankle Surgery.* 1997; 36:322–5.

DCCT Research Group. The effect of intensive treatment of diabetes on the development and progression of long-term complications in insulin-dependent diabetes mellitus. *N Engl J Med* 1993; 329:977-986.

Defronzo RA, Bonadonna RC, Ferrannini E. Pathogenesis of NIDDM: a balanced overview. *Diabetes Care* 1992; 15:318–368.

Delbridge L, Ctercteko G, Fowler C, et al. The aetiology of diabetic neuropathic ulceration of the foot. *British Journal of Surgery* 1985; 72:1-6.

Dhaliwal G, Mukherjee D. Peripheral arterial disease: epidemiology, natural history, diagnosis and treatment. *Int J Angiol* 2007;16:36-44.

Diabetes Technol Ther 2004, 6: 167-177.

Dorresteijn JA, Kriegsman DM, Assendelft WJ, Valk GD. Patient education for preventing diabetic foot ulceration. *Cochrane Database Syst Rev* 2012; CD001488.

Dowd SE, Sun Y, Secor PR, et al. Survey of bacterial diversity in chronic wounds using pyrosequencing, DGGE, and full ribosome shotgun sequencing. *BMC Microbiol* 2008; 8:43.

Du X, Matsumura T, Edelstein D, et al. Inhibition of GAPDH activity by poly (ADP-ribose) polymerase activates three major pathways of hyperglycaemic damage in endothelial cells. *J Clin Investig.* 2003; 112:1049–57.

Ebskov LB. Diabetic amputation and long term survival. *Int.J. Rehab.Res* 1998; 2:403-408.

Edghill EL, Bingham C, Slingerland AS, et al. Hepatocyte nuclear factor-1 beta mutations cause neonatal diabetes and intrauterine growth retardation: Support for a critical role of HNF-1beta in human pancreatic development. *Diabet Med* 2006; 23:1301–1306.

Edmonds ME, Blundell MP, Morris ME, et al. Improved survival of the diabetic foot: The role of a specialized foot clinic. *Q J Med* 1986; 60:763-771.

Edmonds ME, Foster AVM, Saunders EJ. Stage 2: The high risk foot In: A practical Manual of Diabetic Foot care. Blackwell Publishing. 2006 ; 45 (Sep/Oct): 5.

Enne VI, Livermore DM, Stephens P, Hall LM. Persistence of sulphonamide resistance in *Escherichia coli* in the UK despite national prescribing restriction. *Lancet* 2001; 357:1325-8.

Eriksson G, Eklund AE, Kallings LL. The clinical significance of bacterial growth in venous leg ulcers. *Scand J Infect Dis* 1984; 16:175–80.

Faideau B, Larger E, Lepault F, et al. Role of beta-cells in type 1 diabetes pathogenesis. *Diabetes* 2005; 54: S87–96.

Findley K, Oh J, Yang J, et al. Intramural Sequencing Center Comparative Sequencing Program, Kong HH, Segre JA: Topographic diversity of fungal and bacterial communities in human skin. *Nature* 2013, 498**:** 367-370.

Frykberg RG, Armstrong DG, Giurini J, et al. Diabetic foot disorders: a clinical practice guideline. American College of Foot and Ankle Surgeons. *J Foot Ankle Surg* 2000; 39(5 suppl):S1-60.

Frykberg RG, Habershaw GM, Chrzan JS. Epidemiology of the diabetic foot: ulcerations and amputations. In: Contemporary Endocrinology: Clinical Management of Diabetic Neuropathy. edited by Veves A, Humana Press, Totowa, NJ,1998: 273.

Frykberg RG, Larvey L, Pham H, et al. Role of neuropathy and high foot pressures in diabetic foot ulceration. *Diabetes Care* 1998; 21:1714-1719.

Frykberg RG. An evidence-based approach to diabetic foot infections. *Am J Surg* 2003; 186:S44–S54.

Frykberg RG. Epidemiology of the diabetic foot: ulcerations and amputations. *Adv. Wound Care* 1999;12: 139-141.

Frykberg RG. Epidemiology of the diabetic foot: ulcerations and amputations. *Adv. Wound Care* 1999; 12:139-141.

Gadepalli R, Dhawan B, Sreenivas V, et al. A clinico-microbiological study of diabetic foot ulcers in an Indian tertiary care hospital. *Diabetes Care* 2006; 29:1727-1732.

Gaede P, Lund-Andersen H, Parving HH, et al. Effect of a multifactorial intervention on mortality in type 2 diabetes. *N Engl J Med* 2008;358:580–91

Garvey WT. Glucose transport and NIDDM. *Diabetes Care* 1992; 15: 396-410.

Ghadorian SB, Hayati F, Shayanpour S, et al. Diabetes and end-stage renal disease; a review article on new concepts. *J Renal Inj Prev* 2015; 4:28–33.

Gibbons G., Eliopoulos G. M. Infection of the Diabetic Foot. In: Kozak GP, Hoar CS, Rowbotham JL, editors. Management of Diabetic Foot Problems. Philadelphia: WB Saunders; 1984:97–102.

Gillespie KM. Type 1 diabetes: pathogenesis and prevention. *CMAJ* 2006;175:165–170.

Gin H. Infection and diabetes [in French]. *Rev Med Interne* 1993; 14:32–8.

Global Lower Extremity Amputation Study Group: Epidemiology of lower extremity amputation in centres in Europe, North America and East Asia. The Global Lower Extremity Amputation Study Group. *Br J Surg* 2000; 87:328-37.

Gohel MS, et al. The relationship between cytokine concentrations and wound healing in chronic venous ulceration. *J Vasc Surg* 2008; 48:1272–1277.

Gold HS, Moellering Jr RC. Antimicrobial drug resistance. *N Engl J Med* 1996; 335:1445-1453.

Goldberg HJ, Whiteside CI, Fantus IG. The hexosamine pathway regulates the plasminogen activator inhibitor-1 gene promoter and Sp1 transcriptional activation through protein kinase C-beta I and –delta. *J. Biol. Chem* 2002; 277:33833-33841.

Goldstein EJ, Citron DM, Nesbit CA. Diabetic foot infections: bacteriology and activity of 10 oral antimicrobial agents against bacteria isolated from consecutive cases. *Diabetes Care* 1996; 19: 638–41.

Grant DS, Kleimann HK, Goldberg ID, et al. Scatter factor induces blood vessel formation in vivo. *Proc Natl Acad Sci USA* 1993; 90:1937-1941.

Grayson ML, Gibbons GW, Balogh K, et al. Probing to bone in infected pedal ulcers. *JAMA* 1995; 27:721–3.

Guest CB, Park MJ, Johnson DR, Freund GG. The implication of proinflammatory cytokines in type 2 diabetes. *Front Biosci* 2008; 13:5187–5194.

Guillausseau PJ, Meas T, Virally M, et al. Abnormalities in insulin secretion in type 2 diabetes mellitus. *Diabetes and Metabolism* 2008; 34 (Suppl 2) S43–S48.

Gupta A, Gupta R, Sarna M, et al. Prevalence of diabetes, impaired fasting glucose and insulin resistance syndrome in an urban Indian population. *Diabetes Res Clin Pract* 2003; 61:69-76.

Halban PA, Polonsky KS, Bowden DW, et al., β-cell failure in type 2 diabetes: postulated mechanisms and prospects for prevention and treatment. *Diabetes Care* 2014; 37:1751–1758.

Hamalainen H, Ronnemma T, Halonen JP, et al. Factors predicting lower extremity amputations in patients with type 1 or type 2 diabetes mellitus: A population-based 7 year follow-up study. *J Int Med* 1999; 246:97-103

Hampton G, Birke IA. Treatment of wounds caused by pressure and insensitivity. In: Kloth LC, MeCulloch iM, Feeder iA (eds). Wound healing: alternatives in management. Davis, Philadelphia 1990: 196-220.

Hansson C, Hoborn J, Möller A. et al. The microbial flora in venous leg ulcerswithout clinical signs of infection. *Acta Dermato-Venereologica* 1995; 75:24–30.

Harris MI. Diabetes in America: epidemiology and scope of the problem. Diabetes Care 1998; 21(Suppl. 3):C11-C14.

Harris R & Leininger L. Preventive care in rural primary care practice. *Cancer* 1993; 72(3 suppl):1113–1118.

Hart C A, Kariuki S. Antimicrobial resistance in developing countries. *British Medical Journal* 1998; 317, 647–50

Hartemann-Heurtier A, Senneville E. Diabetic foot osteomyelitis. *Diabetes Metab* 2008; 34:87–95.

Hattersley AT & Ashcroft FM. Activating mutations in Kir6.2 and neonatal diabetes: new clinical syndromes, new scientific insights, and new therapy. *Diabetes* 2005; 54, 2503–2513.

Hennis AJJ, Fraser HS, Jonnalagadda R, et al. Explainations for the high risk of diabetes-related amputation in a Carribean population of black African descent and potential for prevention. *Diabetes Care* 2004; 27:2636-2641.

Herath H, Herath R, Wickremasnghie R. Gestational diabetes mellitus and risk of type 2 diabetes 10 years after the index pregnancy in Sri Lankan women-A community based retrospective cohort study. *Plos one* 2017; 12: e0179647.

Hinchliffe RJ, Valk GD, Apelqvist J, et al. A systematic review of the effectiveness of interventions to enhance the healing of chronic ulcers of the foot in diabetes. *Diabetes Metab Res Rev* 2008; 24 (Suppl 1):S119–44.

Hirschl M, Hirschl AM. Bacterial flora in mal perforant and antimicrobial treatment with ceftriaxone. *Chemotherapy* 1992; 38:275–80.

Hokkam EN. Assessment of risk factors in diabetic foot ulceration and their impact on the outcome of the disease. *Primary Care Diabet* 2009; 3: 219-224.

Holt RI. Diagnosis, epidemiology and pathogenesis of diabetes mellitus: an update for psychiatrists. *Br. J. Psychiatry* 2005; (Suppl 47) S55–S63.

Howell-Jones RS, Wilson MJ, Hill KE et al. A review of the microbiology, antibiotic usage and resistance in chronic skin wounds. *J Antimicrob Chemother* 2005; 55:143–9.

Hubner G, Braucle M, Smola H, et al. Differential regulation of pro-inflammatory cytokimes during wound healing in normal and glucocorticoid-treated mice. *Cytokine* 1996; 8:548-556.

Humphrey ARG, Dowse GK, Thomas K, et al. Diabetes and non-traumatic lower extremity amputations: incidence, risk factors and prevention: 12-year follow up study in Nauru. *Diabetes Care* 1996; 19:710–714.

Humphrey LL, Palumbo PJ, Butters MA, et al. The contribution of non-insulin dependent diabetes to lower extremity amputation in the communit. *Arch. Intern. Med* 1994; 154:885-892.

Jalava J, Skurnik M, Toivanen A, et al. Bacterial PCR in the diagnosis of joint infection. *Ann Rheum Dis* 2001; 60:287–9.

Jeffcoate WJ. The incidence of amputation in diabetes. *Acta Chir Beig* 2005; 105:140-144

Jones V. Debridement of diabetic foot lesions. *The Diabetic Foot* 1998;1:88–94.

Joseph WS & Tan JS. Infections in diabetic foot ulcerations. *Curr Infect Dis Rep* 2003; 5:391–7.

Joseph WS, Axler DA. Microbiology and antimicrobial therapy of diabetic foot infections. *Clin Podiatr Med Surg* 1990; 7: 467–81.

Joseph WS, Axler DA. Microbiology and antimicrobial therapy of diabetic foot infections. *Clin Podiatr Med Surg* 1990; 7:467–81.

Joshi N, Caputo G, Weitekamp M, et al. Infections in patients with diabetes mellitus. *N Engl J Med* 1999; 341:1906–12.

Joshi SR & Parikh RM. India - diabetes capital of the world: now heading towards hypertension. *J Assoc Physicians India* 2007; 55:323-4.

Kahn SE, Andrikopoulos S, Verchere CB. Islet amyloid: a long-recognised but underappreciated pathological feature of type 2 diabetes. *Diabetes* 1999; 48: 241-253

Kannel WB, McGee DL. Diabetes and cardiovascular disease: the Framingham study. *JAMA* 1979; 241:2035-2038.

Kissebah AH, Vydelingum N, Murray R, et al. Relation of body fat distribution to metabolic complications of obesity. *Clin Enidocrinol Metab* 1982; 54:254-60.

Kiziltan ME., Gunduz A, Kiziltan G, et al. Study of peripheral neuropathy in patients with diabetic foot ulcers: clinical and nerve conduction study. *J Neurol Sci* 2007; 258:75-9.

Klein R, Klein BEK, Moss SE, et al. The Wisconsin Epidemiologic Study of Diabetic Retinopathy, XVII: the 14-year incidence and progression of diabetic retinopathy and associated risk factors in type I diabetes. *Ophthalmology* 1998; 105:1801–1815.

Knox CM, Cevellos V, Dean D. 16S ribosomal DNA typing for identification of pathogens in patients with bacterial keratitis. *J. Clin. Microbiol* 1998; 36:3492–3496.

Koya D, Jirousek MR, Lin YW et al. Characterization of protein kinase C beta isoform activation on the gene expression of transforming growth factor-beta extracellular matrix components and prostanoids in the glomeruli of diabetic rats *J. Clin Invest* 1997; 100:115-126.

Krosnick, A. The diabetes and obesity epidemic among the Pima Indians. *N J Med* 2000; 97:31–3.

Kumar A, Goel MK, Jain RB, Khanna P, Chaudhary V. India towards diabetes control: Key issues. *Australas Med J* 2013; 6:524-31.

LaingSP, SwerdlowAJ, SlaterSD, et al. Mortality from heart disease in a cohort of 23,000 patients with insulin-treated diabetes. *Diabetologia* 2003: 46:760-765.

Larsson J, Apleqvist J, Agardh CD, et al. Decreasing incidence of major amputation in diabetic patients: a consequence of a multidisciplinary foot care team approach? *Diabetic Med* 1995; 12:770-776.

Larvey LA, Armstrong DG, Vela S, et al. Practical criteria for screening patients at high risk for diabetic foot ulceration. *Arch. Intern. Med* 1998; 158:157-162.

Larvey LA, Ashry HR, Van Houtum W, et al. Variation in the incidence and proportion of diabetes-related amputations in minorities. *Diabetes Care* 1996; 19: 48-52.

Lavery LA, Armstrong DG, Wunderlich RP, et al. Risk factors for foot infection in person with diabetes. *Diabetes Care* 2006; 6:1288-1293.

Lavigne JP, Sotto A, Dunyach-Remy C., et al. New molecular techniques to study the skin microbiota of diabetic foot ulcers. *Adv Wound Care* 2014; 4:38-49.

Leahy JL, Bonner-Weir S, Weir GC. β- cell dysfunction induced by chronic hyperglycaemia. *Diabetes Care* 1992; 15: 443–451.

Lee JS, Lu M, Lee VS, et al. Lower extremity amputation. Incidence, risk factors, and mortality in the Oklahoma Indian Diabetes Study. *Diabetes* 1993; 42:876-882.

Lehto S, Pyorala K, Ronnemaa T, et al. Risk fators predicting lower extremity amputation in NIDDM. *Diabetes Care* 1996; 196:607-612.

Lehto S, Pyorala K, Ronnemaa T, et al. Risk fators predicting lower extremity amputation in NIDDM. *Diabetes Care* 1996; 19:607-612.

Leon BM, Maddox TM. Diabetes and cardiovascular disease: epidemiology, biological mechanisms, treatment recommendations and future research. World J *Diabetes* 2015;6:1246–1258.

Levey AS, Stevens LA, Schmid CH, et al. A newequation to estimate glomerular filtration rate. *Ann Intern Med* 2009; 150:604–12.

Levin A, Hemmelgarn B, Culleton B, et al. Guidelines for the management of chronic kidney disease. *CMAJ* 2008; 179:1154–62.

Lillioja S, Mott D, Spraul M, et al. Insulin resistance and insulin secretory dysfunction as precursors of non-insulin-dependent diabetes mellitus *N Engl J Med* 1993; 329:1988-1992.

Lilly EL, Halanych KM, Anderson DM. Species boundaries and global biogeography of the *Alexandrium tamarense* complex (Dinophyceae). *J. Phycol* 2007; 43:1329-1338.

Lin HV, Ren H, Samuel VT, et al. Diabetes in mice with selective impairment of insulin action in Glut4-expressing tissues. *Diabetes* 2011:60:700–709.

Lipsky BA, Aragón-Sánchez J, Diggle M, et al. IWGDF Guidance on the diagnosis and management of foot infections in persons with diabetes. *Diabetes Metab Res Rev* 2015.

Lipsky BA, Berendt AR, Deery HG, et al. Diagnosis and treatment of diabetic foot infections. *Clin. Infect. Dis* 2004; 39: 885-910.

Lipsky BA, McDonald D, Litka PA. Treatment of infected diabetic foot ulcers: Topical MSI-78 vs. oral ofloxacin (abstract) *Diabetologia* 1997; 40:482.

Lipsky BA, Pecoraro RE, Larson SA, et al. Outpatient management of uncomplicated lower-extremity infections in diabetic patients. *Arch. Intern. Med* 1990; 150:790-797.

Lipsky BA, Peters EJ, Berendt AR et al. International Working Group on Diabetic Foot: specific guidelines for the treatment of diabetic foot infections. *Diabetes Metab Res Rev* 2011; 2012 (28) Suppl. (1)):234–5.

Lipsky BA. Evidence-based antibiotic therapy of diabetic foot infections FEMS. *Immunol Med Microbiol* 1999; 26: 267–76.

Louie TJ, Bartlett JG, Tally FP, et al. Aerobic and anaerobic bacteria in diabetic foot ulcers. *Ann Intern Med* 1976; 85:461-463.

Mackowiak PA, Jones SR, Smith JW. Diagnostic value of sinus-tract cultures in chronic osteomyelitis. *J Am Med Assoc* 1978; 239:2772–5.

Maillard LC. Action des acides amines sur les sucres: formation des melanoidines par voie methodique. *C R Hebd Seances Acad Sci* 1912a; 154:66–68.

Martin JM, Zenilman JM, Lazarus GS. Molecular microbiology: new dimensions for cutaneous biology and wound healing. *J Invest Dermatol* 2010; 130:38–48.

Marvaso A, Esposito S, Noviello S. Outpatient parenteral antibiotic therapy (OPAT) of diabetic foot infections with piperacillin/tazobactam. *Infez Med* 2002; 10:230–5.

Mayfield JA, Reiber GE, Nelson RG, et al. A foot risk classification system to predict diabetic amputation in Pima Indians. *Diabetes Care* 1996; 19:704-709.

Mayfield JA, Reiber GE, Nelson RG, et al. A foot risk classification system to predict diabetic amputation in Pima Indians. *Diabetes Care* 1996; 19:704-709.

Mayfield JA, Sugarman JR: The use of Semmes-Weinstein monofilament and other threshold tests for preventing foot ulceration and amputation in people with diabetes. *J Fam Pract* 2000; 49 (Suppl.):517–529.

Melendez JH, Frankel YM, An AT, et al. Real-time PCR assays compared to culture-based approaches for identification of aerobic bacteria in chronic wounds. Clin *Microbiol Infect* 2010; 16: 1762–9.=

Menon VU, Kumar KV, Gilchrist A, et al. Prevalence of known and undetected diabetes and associated risk factors in central Kerala - ADEPS. *Diabetes Res Clin Pract* 2006; 74:289-94.

Mohan V, Sandeep S, Deepa R, Shah B, Varghese C. Epidemiology of type 2 diabetes: Indian scenario. *Indian J Med Res* 2007; 125:217-230.

Monson JP, Koios G, Toms GC, et al., Relationship between retinopathy and glycemic control in insulin-dependent and non-insulin-dependent diabetes. *J R Soc Med* 1986; 79:274-276.

Moore SA, Peterson RG, Felten DL et al., A quantitative comparison of motor and sensory conduction velocities in short- and long-term streptozotocin- and alloxan-diabetic rats. *J Neurol Sci* 1980; 48:133–152.

Mooy J, Grootenhuis P, de Vries H, et al. Prevalence and determinants of glucose intolerance in a Dutch Caucasian population: the Hoorn study. *Diabetes Care* 1995; 18:1270–1273.

Moss SE, Klein R, Klein B. The prevalence and incidence of lower extremity amputation in a diabetic population. *Arch. Intern. Med* 1992; 152: 610-616.

Moss SE, Klein R, Klein BEK. Cause-specific mortality in a population-based study of diabetes. *Am J Public Health* 1991; 81:1158-1162 CDCP 2003.

Muller IS, De Grauw WJ, Van Gerwen WH, et al. Foot ulceration and lower limb amputation in type 2 diabetic patients in Dutuch primary health care. *Diabetes Care* 2002; 25:570-574.

Murea M, Ma L, Freedman BI. Genetic and environmental factors associated with type 2 diabetes and diabetic vascular complications. *Rev Diabetic Stud RDS* 2012; 9:6-22.

Murray HJ, Young MJ, Hollis S, et al. The association between callus formation, high pressures and neuropathy in diabetic foot ulceration. *Diabet Med* 1996; 13:979-982.

Musa H, Ahmed M: Associated risk factors and management of chronic diabetic foot ulcers exceeding 6 months' duration. *Diabet Foot Ankle* 2012, 3:1–6.

Nelson RG, Gohdes DM, Everhart JE, et al. Lower extremity amputations in NIDDM: 12-yr follow up study in Pima Indians. *Diabetes Care* 1988; 11:8-16.

Nielsen JV. Peripheral neuropathy, hypertension, foot ulcers and amputation among Saudi Arabian patients with type 2 diabetes. *Diabetes Res Clin Pract* 1998; 41:63-69.

Noble JA & Erlich HA. Genetics of type 1 diabetes. Cold Spring Harb Perspect Med 2 2012; a007732.

Noor S, Zubair M, Ahmad J. Diabetic foot ulcer–a review on pathophysiology, classification, and microbial etiology. *Diabetes Metab. Syndr* 2015; 9:192–199.

Nyenwe EA, Jerkins TW, Umpierrez GE, et al., Management of type 2 diabetes: evolving strategies for the treatment of patients with type 2 diabetes. *Metabolism* 2011; 60:1–23

Oyibo SO, Jude EB, Tarawneh I, et al. A comparison of two diabetic foot ulcer classification systems: the Wagner and the university of Texas wound classification systems. *Diabetes Care* 2001; 24:84–8.

Palumbo PJ, Melton LJI. Peripheral vascular disease and diabetes. In National Diabetes Data Group(ed): Diabetes In America, 2nd ed (NIH publ. no. 495-1468). Washington, DC, U.S. Government Printing Office. 1995:401-408.

Paniagua JA. Nutrition, insulin resistance and dysfunctional adipose tissue determine the different components of metabolic syndrome. *World J Diabetes* 2016 15;7:483-514.

Papanas N, Eleftheriadou I, Tentolouris N, Maltezos E. Advances in the topical treatment of diabetic foot ulcers. *Curr Diabetes Rev* 2012; 8:209–18.

Parisi MC, Zantut-Wittmann DE, Pavin EJ et al. Comparison of three systems of classification in predicting the outcome of diabetic foot ulcers in Brazilian population. Eur J Endocrinol. 2008; 159:417–22.

Park JE, Barbul A. understanding the role of immune regulation in wound healing. *Am J Surg* 2004; 187:11S-16S.

Parkhouse N, Le Quesne PM. Impaired neurogenic vascular response in patients with diabetes and neuropathic foot lesions. *N. Engl. J. Med* 1988; 318:1306.

Partanen J, Niskanen L, Lehtinen J, et al. Natural history of peripheral neuropathy in patients with non-insulin-dependent diabetes mellitus. *N Engl J Med* 1995; 333:89–94.

Patel P, Abate N. Body fat distribution and insulin resistance. *Nutrients* 2013; 5:2019–2027.

Patrick R. Murray, Ellen Jo Baron, James H. Jorgensen, Marie Louise Landry, Michael A. Pfaller, Manual of Clinical Microbiology, 9th ed., 2007: American Society of Microbiology Washington, DC.

Pecoraro RE, Reiber G, Burgess EM. Pathways to diabetic limb amputation: basis for prevention. *Diabetes Care* 1990; 13:513.

Pendergrass M, Bertoldo A, Bonadonna R, et al., Muscle glucose transport and phosphorylation in type 2 diabetic, obese non-diabetic, and genetically predisposed individuals. *Am J Physiol Endocrinol Metab* 2007; 292:E92–E100.

Pendsey S. Epidemiological aspects of diabetic foot. *J Diabetes Develop Countries* 1994; 2: 37-38.

Peters EJ, Lavery LA. Effectiveness of the diabetic foot risk classification system of the international working group on the diabetic foot. *Diabetes Care* 2001; 24:1442–7.

Peterson RG. Animal Models of Diabetes. Harwood Academic Publishers: Amsterdam; 2001.

Peterson RG. Animal Models of Diabetes: A primer. Harwood Academic Publisher; Newark, NJ. The Zucker Diabetic Fatty Rat. 2000.

Pongsachareonnont P, Honglertnapakul W, Chatsuwan T. Comparison of methods for identifying causative bacterial microorganisms in presumed acute endophthalmitis: conventional culture, blood culture, and PCR. *BMC Infect Dis* 2017; 17: 165

Price LB, Liu CM, Melendez JH, et al. Community analysis of chronic wound bacteria using 16S rRNA gene-based pyrosequencing: impact of diabetes and antibiotics on chronic wound microbiota. *PLoS One* 2009:e6462.

Prompers L, Schaper N, Apelqvist J, et al. Prediction of outcome in individuals with diabetic foot ulcers: focus on the differences between individuals with and without peripheral arterial disease. The EURODIALE Study. *Diabetologia* 2008; 51:747–55.

Pugliese G, Pricci F, Pugliese F *et al*. Mechanism of glucose enhanced extracellular matrix accumulation in rat glomerular mesangial cells. *Diabetes* 1994; 43:478-490.

Raja NS. Microbiology of diabetic foot infections in a teaching hospital in Malaysia: a retrospective study of 194 cases. J Microbiol Immuno Infect 2007; 40:39-44.

Raja NS. Microbiology of diabetic foot infections in a teaching hospital in Malaysia: a retrospective study of 194 cases. *J Microbiol Immuno Infect* 2007; 40:39-44.

Ramachandran A, Snehalatha C, Kapur A et al. High prevalence of diabetes and impaired glucose tolerance in India: National Urban Diabetes Survey. *Diabetologia* 2001; 44:1094–1101.

Ramachandran A. Specific problems of the diabetic foot in developing countries. *Diabetes Metab Res Rev* 2004; 20:S19–22.

Ramakant P, Verma AK, Misra R, et al. Changing microbiological profile of pathogenic bacteria in diabetic foot infections: time for a rethink on which empirical therapy to choose? *Diabetologia* 2011; 54: 58–64.

Ramsey SD, Newton K, Blough D et al. Incidence, outcomes and costs of foot ulcers in patients with diabetes. *Diabetes Care* 1999; 22:382–7.

Rask-Madsen C, King GL. Vascular complications of diabetes: mechanisms of injury and protective factors. *Cell Metab* 2013; 17:20–33.

Rathur HM, Boulton HJ. The diabetic foot. *Clin Dermatol* 2007; 25:109–20.

Raymakers JT, Houben AJ, et al. The effect of diabetes and severe ischaemia on the penetration of ceftazidime into tissues of the limb. *Diabetic Medicine* 2001; 18: 229-234.

Reed JF. An audit of lower extremity complications in octogenarian patients with diabetes mellitus. *Int J Low Extrem Wounds* 2004; 3:161–4.

Reiber GE, Bokyo EJ, Smith DG. Lower extremity foot ulcers and amputations in diabetes. In National Diabetes Data Group (ed): Diabetes in America, 2nd ed

(NIH publ. no.95 1468). Washington, DC, U.S. Government Printing Office: 1995:409-428.

Reiber GE, Lipsky BA, Gibbons GW. The burden of diabetic foot ulcers. *Am J Surg* 1998; 176(Suppl 2A):S5–10.

Reiber GE, Pecoraro RE, Koepsell TD. Risk factors for amputation in patients with diabetes mellitus: a case control study. *Ann Intern Med* 1992; 117:97–105.

Reiber GE, Vileikyte L, Boyko EJ, et al. Causal pathways for incident lower extremity ulcers in patients with diabetes from two settings. *Diabetes Care* 1999; 22:157-162.

Reiber GE. The epidemiology of diabetic foot problems. *Diabet Med* 1996;13:(suppl 1) S6-S11.

Reinehr T. Type 2 diabetes mellitus in children and adolescents. *World J Diabetes* 2013; 4:270–28.

Resnick HE, Carter EA, Sosenko JM, et al. Incidence of lower extremity amputation in American Indians: The Strong Heart Study. *Diabetes Care* 2004; 27:1885-1891.

Resnick HE, Valsania P, Phillips CL. Diabetes mellitus and non-traumatic lower extremity amputation in black and white Americans: The national health and nutrition examination survey epidemiological follow-up study, 1971-1992. *Arch Intern Med* 1999; 159:2470-2475.

Resnick HE, Valsania P, Phillips CL. Diabetes mellitus and non-traumatic lower extremity amputation in black and white Americans: The national health and nutrition examination survey epidemiological follow-up study, 1971-1992. *Arch Intern Med* 1999; 159:2470-2475.

Richmond W. Scand J Clin Lab Invest 1972; 29(Suppl 26), Abstract 3: 25.

Roberts WC: The Friedewald-Levy-Fredrickson formula for calculating low-density lipoprotein cholesterol, the basis for lipid-lowering therapy. *Am J Cardiol* 1988, 62: 345-346.

Robinson LR, Stolov WC, Rubner DE, et al. Height is an independent risk factor for neuropathy in diabetic men. *Diabetes Res Clin Pract* 1992; 16:97-102.

Sadikot SM, Nigam A, Das S, et al. The burden of diabetes and impaired fasting glucose in India using the WHO 1999 critetia. Prevalence of diabetes in India study (PODIS). On behalf of Diabetes India. *Diabetes Research and Clinical Practice* 2004; 66: 301-307.

Sapico FL, Witte JL, Canawati HN, et al. The infected foot of the diabetic patient:quantitative microbiology Guidelines for Diabetic Foot Infections CID 2004:39 (1 October) 905 and analysis of clinical features. *Rev Infect Dis* 1984; 6(Suppl 1): S171 6.

Schabereiter-Gurtner C, Maca S, Rolleke S, et al. 16S rDNA–based identification of bacteria from conjunctival swabs by PCR and DGGE fingerprinting. *Invest Ophthalmol Vis Sci*, 2001.

Schraibman IG. The significance of beta-haemolytic streptococci in chronic leg ulcers. Annals of the Royal College of Surgeons of England 1990; 72: 123–124.

Schubert S, Heesemann J. Infections in diabetes mellitus [in German]. *Immun Infekt* 1995; 23:200–204.

Schultz GS, Sibbald RG, Falanga V, et al. Wound bed preparation: a systematic approach to wound management. *Wound Repair Regen* 2003; 11(Suppl 1):S1–28.

Selby JV, Karter AJ, Ackerson LM, et al. Developing a prediction rule from automated clinical database to identify high-risk patients in a large population with diabetes. *Diabetes Care* 2001; 24:1547-1555.

Selby ZV, Zhang D. Risk factors for lower extremity amputation in persons with diabetes. *Diabetes Care* 1995; 18: 509-516.

Serra MB, Barroso WA, da Silva NN et al. From inflammation to current and alternative therapies involved in wound healing. *International Journal of Inflammation* 2017; 34:15-17.

Shah BR, Hux JE. Quantifying the risk of infectious diseases for people with diabetes. *Diabetes Care* 2003; 26: 510-513.

Sharma VS, Khadka PB, Joshi A, Sharma R: Common pathogens isolated in diabetic foot infection in Bir Hospital. *Kathmandu University Medical Journal* 2006, 4: 295-30.

Shaw JE, Sicree RA, Zimmet PZ. Global estimates of the prevalence of diabetes for 2010 and 2030. *Diabetes Res Clin Pract* 2010; 87:4–14.

Shihabi Z K, Konen J C, O'Connor M L. Albuminuria vs urinary total protein for detecting chronic renal disorders. *Clin. Chem* 1991; 37:621–624.

Shimomura I, et al. Insulin selectively increases SREBP-1c mRNA in livers of rats with streptozotocin-induced diabetes. *Proc Natl Acad Sci USA* 1999; 96:13656–13661.

Simpson DM, Ross R. Effects of heterologous antineutrophil serum in guinea pigs. Hematologic and ultrastructural observations. *Am J Pathol* 1971; 65:79–102.

Smith K, Collier A, Townsend EM, et al. One step closer to understanding the role of bacteria in diabetic foot ulcers: characterising the microbiome of ulcers. *BMC Microbiol* 2016;16:54

Sohn MW, Stuck RM, Pinzur M, et al. Lower-extremity amputation risk after charcotarthropathy and diabetic foot ulcer. *Diabetes Care* 2010; 33: 98–100.

Songini M, Lombardo C. The Sardinian way to type 1 diabetes. *Journal of Diabetes Science and Technology* 2010; 4:1248–1255.

Sosenko JM, Gladia MT, Fournier AM et al. Body stature as a risk factor for diabetic sensory neuropathy. *Am J Med* 1986; 80:1031-1034.

Sotto A, Lina G, Richard JL, Combescure C, Bourg G, Vidal L, et al. Virulence potential of Staphylococcus aureus strains isolated from diabetic foot ulcers: a new paradigm. *Diabetes Care* 2008; 31:2318–24.

Speers DJ. Clinical applications of molecular biology for infectious diseases. *Clin Biochem Rev* 2006; 27:39-51.

Stess RM, Jensen SR, Mirmiran R. The role of dynamic planter pressures in diabetic foot ulcers. *Diabetes Care* 1997; 20:855-858.

Steven PM, William RH: Peripheral Arterial Disease in Patients With Diabetes: *Journal of the American College of Cardiology* 2006; 47:5.

Stevens MJ, Goss DE, Foster AVM, et al. Abnormal digital pressure measurements in diabetic neuropathic foot ulceration. *Diabetic Med* 1993; 10:909-915.

Sugiuchi H, Uji Y, Okabe H, et al. Direct measurement of high-density lipoprotein cholesterol in serum with polyethylene glycol-modified enzymes and sulfated alpha-cyclodextrin. *Clin Chem* 1995; 41:717–23.

Tallapragada DSP, Karpe PA, Tikoo K. Long-lasting partnership between insulin resistance and endothelial dysfunction: role of metabolic memory. *Br J Pharmacol* 2015; 172:4012–4023.

Tan JS, Friedman NM, Hazelton-Miller C, et al. Can aggressive treatment of diabetic foot infection reduce the need for above-ankle amputation? *Clin Infect Dis* 1996; 23: 286-291.

Tentolouris N, Al-Sabbagh S, Walker MG, et al. Mortality in diabetic and nondiabetic patients after amputations performed from 1990 to 1995: a year follow up study. *Diabetes Care* 2004; 27:1598-1604.

Tesfaye T, Shikur B, Shimels T, et al. *BMC Endocr Disord* 2016; 16:68.

The International Working Group on the Diabetic Foot. The International Consensus on the Diabetic Foot. The International Working Group on the Diabetic Foot, Amsterdam, Netherlands 1999.

Thiruvoipati T, Kielhorn CE, Armstrong EJ. Peripheral artery disease in patients with diabetes: Epidemiology, mechanisms, and outcomes. *World J Diabetes* 2015; 6:961–969.

Thompson DE. The effects of mechanical stress on soft tissue. 1988; In: The diabetic foot, Levin ME, O'Neil LW (eds) ed 4., CV Mosby, St. Louis: 83.

Tomlinson DR. Future prevention and treatment of diabetic neuropathy. *Diabetes Metab* 1998; 24(Suppl 3):79–83.

Trautner C, Hasstert B, Giani G, et al. Incidence of lower limb amputations and diabetes. *Diabetes Care* 1996; 19:1006-1009.

Umpierrez GE, Casals MM, Gebhart SP, et al. Diabetic ketoacidosis in obese African-Americans. Diabetes 1995; 44:790–795.

United Kingdom Prospective Diabetes Study Group (UKPDS). Intensive blood glucose control with sulfonylureas or insulin compared with conventional treatment and risk of complications in patients with type 2 diabetes (UKPDS). *Lancet* 1998; 352:837-853

Urakami T, Habu M, Kuwabara R, et al. Insulin resistance at diagnosis in Japanese children with type 2 diabetes mellitus. Pediatrics international: official journal of the Japan Pediatric Society. 2012 [Epub ahead of print] Retrospective chart review of 160 Japanese children diagnosed with T2DM by standard screening program. IR was found in all patients, increasing with increasing BMI.

Urbancic Rovan C, Gubina M., Infection in superficial diabetic foot ulcers. *Clinc Infect Disease* 1997; 25:S184-5.

Valones MA , Guimarães RL , Brandão LA , et al. Principles and applications of polymerase chain reaction in medical diagnostic fields: a review. *Braz J Microbiol* 2009; 40:1–11.

Veves A, Murray H, Young MJ, et al. Do high foot pressures lead to foot ulcerations?: A prospective study [abstract]. *Diabetologia* 1991; 34:A40.

Viswanathan V, Jasmine JJ, Snehalatha C, et al. Prevalence of pathogens in diabetic foot infection in south Indian type 2 diabetic patients. *JAPI* 2002; 50:1013-1016.

Viswanathan V, Kumpatla S. Indian Diabetic Amputation Study Group. Patterns and causes of amputation in diabetic patients: A multicentre study from India. *JAPI* 2011; 59:148-151.

Wagner FW: The dysvascular foot: a system of diagnosis and treatment. *Foot Ankle* 1981; 2:64 -122.

Wall IB, Davies CE, Hill KE, et al. Potential role of anaerobic cocci in impaired human wound healing. *Wound Repair Regen* 2002; 10:346-353.

Weigelt C, Rose B, Poschen U, et al. Immune mediators in patients with acute diabetic foot syndrome. *Diabetes Care* 2009; 32:1491–149.

Weir MR. Microalbuminuria and cardiovascular disease. *Clin J Am Soc Nephrol* 2007; 2:581-590.

Weiss J, Dimpfel W, Schröder JM. Nerve conduction changes and fine structural alterations of extra- and intrafusal muscle and nerve fibers in streptozotocin diabetic rats. *Muscle Nerve* 1995;18:175–184.

Weitz JI, Byrne J, Clagett GP, et al. Diagnosis and treatment of chronic arterial insufficiency of the lower extremities: A critical review. *Circulation* 1996; 94: 3026–49

Wendland EM, Torloni MR, Falavigna M, et al. Gestational diabetes and pregnancy outcomes—a systematic review of the World Health Organization (WHO) and the International Association of Diabetes in Pregnancy Study Groups (IADPSG) diagnostic criteria. *BMC Pregnancy Childbirth* 2012;12:23.

Wheat LJ, Allen SD, Henry, et al. Diabetic foot infections: Bacteriologic analysis. *Arch Intern Med* 1986; 146:1935-1940.

Whiting DR, Guariguata L, Weil C, et al. IDF diabetes atlas: global estimates of the prevalence of diabetes for 2011 and 2030. *Diabetes Res Clin Pract* 2011; 94:311–21.

Wilcox G. Insulin and insulin resistance. *Clin Biochem Rev* 2005;26:19–39.

Wild S, Roglic G, Green A, et al. Global prevalence of diabetes: Estimates for the year 2000 and projections for 2030. *Diabetes Care* 2004. 27: 1047–1053.

Williams DT, Hilton JR, et al. Diagnosing foot infection in diabetes. *Clin Infect Dis* 2004, 39: S83-S86.

Williams KJ, Tabas I. The response-to-retention hypothesis of early atherogenesis. *Arterioscler Thromb Vasc Biol* 1995; 15:551–61.

Witte MB, Barbul A. General principles of wound healing. *Surg Clin North Am* 1997; 77:509-528.

Yajnik C, et al. FTO gene variants are strongly associated with type 2 diabetes in South Asian Indians. *Diabetologia* 2009; 52, 247–252.

Yamagata K, Furuta H, Oda N, et al. Mutations in the hepatocyte nuclear factor-4α gene in maturity- onset diabetes of the young (MODY1). *Nature* 1996; 384:458–460.

Yoshida M, Akaike T, Wada Y, et al. Therapeutic effects of imidazolineoxyl N-oxide against endotoxin shock through its direct nitric oxide-scavenging activity. *Biochem Biophys Res Commun* 1994; 202:923-930.

Zargar AH, Khan AK, Masoodi SR, et al. Prevalence of type 2 diabetes mellitus and impaired glucose tolerance in the Kashmir Valley of the Indian subcontinent. *Diabetes Res Clin Pract* 2000; 47:135-6.

Zochodone DW: Diabetic polyneuropathy: an update. *Curr Opin Neurol* 2008; 21:527–533.

Zubair M, Malik A, Ahmad J. Clinico-bacteriology and risk factors for the diabetic foot infection with multidrug resistant microorganisms in North India. *Biol Med* 2010; 2: 22–34

www.ingramcontent.com/pod-product-compliance
Lightning Source LLC
LaVergne TN
LVHW082338200926
848481LV00012B/3381
* 9 7 9 8 2 3 1 0 1 3 8 0 7 *